DEDICATION

This book is dedicated with eternal gratitude
to
CHARAN SINGH

The Humpty Dumpty Syndrome

Lift Yourself
From Back Pain
Without Drugs or Surgery

Harry S. Oxenhandler, M.D.
Diplomate in Acupuncture NCCAOM

The Humpty Dumpty Syndrome
Lift Yourself From Back Pain Without Drugs or Surgery

by Harry S. Oxenhandler, M.D.
    Diplomate in Acupuncture NCCAOM

Published by: Master's Plan Publishing L.L.C.
               2727 NW Ninth Street
               Corvallis, OR 97330
Website: http://www.mastersplanpublishing.com

Library of Congress Control Number: 2003090567
ISBN: 0-9727736-0-6
Printed in the United States of America
0 9 8 7 6 5 4 3 2 1

DISCLAIMER

The purpose of this book is to **educate** both laypersons and health care professionals about pelvic tilt/short leg syndrome. Do not consider the information given in this book as providing medical treatment. I am not establishing a physician-patient relationship. The principles and techniques described in this book are sound, tried and true and every effort has been make to ensure that the information in this book is correct. But, there may be mistakes, both typographical and in content. The person with chronic low back pain is strongly advised to seek the help of a skilled and experienced health care professional in the search for a pain-free lower back. Let him/her help you through the methods and techniques offered in this book.

THE AUTHOR AND THE PUBLISHING COMPANY SHALL HAVE NEITHER LIABILITY NOR RESPONSIBILITY TO ANY PERSON OR ENTITY WITH RESPECT TO ANY INJURY OR DAMAGE CAUSED OR ALLEGED TO HAVE BEEN CAUSED, DIRECTLY OR INDIRECTLY, BY THE INFORMATION CONTAINED IN THIS BOOK.

THANK YOU

to the teachers and mentors of my professional life, because of whose timely advice, help, friendship, love and inspiration, my direction became clear, my burden lighter and my journey more pleasant.

Charan Singh; Gurinder Singh; Louis and Bertha Oxenhandler; Lucy Ludwig Oxenhandler; Gary Oxenhandler; Alan Oxenhandler; John, Jacob and Anne Oxenhandler; Clara and Oscar Sandweiss; Miss Batterton; Dorothy Louise Chestnut; Stan London, M.D.; Wallace Klein; Sam Covell, PhD.; Norton Kalishman, M.D.; Larry Laycob, M.D.; Harry Mittelman, M.D.; Jill Eichengreen; Steve Samuels; Bob Suffian; Maury Abramson; Harry C. Raiffie; Herb Goldberg, PhD.; Fred Lucas, M.D.; Nathan Galloway, M.D.; Jeff Mishell, M.D.; Miriam Lee, O.M.D.; Paramahansa Yogananda; Harold and Bertha Plume; Michael Jacobs,M.D.;Vicki Jones; Arvis Justi; John Clarke, M.D.; Darla Wolgast; Donna Bosser; Valerie Bridwell Cannon; Carrie Lonnquist; The one and only Connie Allen; Todd Brown; Rick Rosetta; Len Mcbride, D.C.; Ian Duncan, M.D.; Philip Greenman, D.O.; Ed Stiles, D.O.; Robert Ward, D.O.; Mitch Ellkiss, D.O.; Neal Gladstone; Ed Hurst; Holly Peterson; Fred Hirsh, M.D.; Howard Korn, M.D.; Grand Master Hyong Kyun Shin; Suzanne Rushman; the friendly and talented people at Family Shoe Service.

ACKNOWLEDGMENTS

This book is the result of a collaborative effort. Help came from many sources. Thank you all very much.

My wife, Lucy, who gave me the time, the encouragement and the support; my children, John, Jacob and Anne, Mom and Dad, my brothers, Gary and Alan for the love and support; Doug Bloch for the initial inspiration; Barbara Baldwin for the initial scrutiny of the manuscript and the encouragement to continue; Marilyn Schwader at clarityofvision.com for a great job of editing and for encouragement and support. Alan Oxenhandler for help with the design and graphics; Holly Peterson at Ball Studio for the author's photograph; Tom Lindberg and Kate Johnson for the outstanding graphics and timely and friendly manner in which it was done. Dan Poynter at ParaPublishing for suggestions and for turning me on to One-On-One Book Production and Marketing, Carolyn Porter and Alan Gadney—who brought the book to life and worked the magic to make it all happen; Faye Kimball who told me years ago that I would write this book; Margie Dilson for her friendship, her insightful advice and her beautiful being; Dan Dutey for the illustrations; Peter Sears for being the taskmaster and cheerleader; Connie Allen for the love and support; Linda Courtney for reading the early manuscript and encouraging me to continue; **a special thank you to all of my dear patients who have entrusted me with their health and given me much experience, wisdom and love.**

TABLE OF CONTENTS

FOREWORD

Dear Reader,

Some years ago, I became quite ill. I developed a condition known as "tic doloreaux" (pronounced "tick dough-low-roo"). This is a problem in which the fifth cranial nerve in the brain fires erratically, unexpectedly and spontaneously, causing an extremely painful sensation to shoot across the face. This condition lasted nearly three years and resulted in my having two brain operations within a period of three weeks. Three years later, I had another attack and another kind of operation to deaden the nerve to that part of my face. I am well now, thank God.

I tell you this because as a result of this illness, I am much more sensitive to the suffering of others than I have ever been in my life. I have an understanding of pain that I otherwise would not have. I know what pain is, how it can torture the mind and body, and what joy it is to finally get relief. In retrospect, this understanding was a blessing in disguise. After that illness, I began to focus my medical practice on the treatment of painful conditions.

Life is very difficult. Human suffering takes many forms and no one can say that one person's pain or that one kind of pain is worse than another. However, *physical* pain, if not the worst kind of pain, is certainly among the top two on my misery list. Certainly it is one of the most common reasons that people go to the doctor. In fact, of all the different kinds of physical pain that exist, low back pain is the second most common reason for visiting the doctor.

Low back pain affects approximately *80 percent of all adults* at one time or another. Yes, you read that correctly! Eighty percent of all adults! The yearly cost of the treatment of low back pain is absolutely astounding (in the billions!) and this does not even include the amount of money in lost wages from the disability of workers. But the purpose of this book is *not* to tell you about the socioeconomics of low back pain. I'm going to tell you how to get rid of it.

There are two kinds of low back pain: acute and chronic. Acute low back pain lasts for less than six weeks. This type of pain is usually the result of an injury of some sort, such as the low back strain that may occur from having worked too long in the garden or from having lifted something a little too heavy. This type of low back problem, although very uncomfortable, is easily treatable with bed rest, muscle relaxant medication and analgesics (pain medication). Even without *any* treatment, it usually gets better within 30 days. A faster way to get rid of it is with spinal manipulation or acupuncture.

The second type of low back pain is chronic low back pain. Chronic low back pain lasts for longer than six weeks—often for many years—and is completely different. There are two types of chronic low back pain: surgically treatable and non-surgically treatable, or medical, low back pain. By far, the most common type of low back pain is medical back pain. There are *millions* of people in the United States alone that are living with chronic medical low back pain.

Chronic, medical low back pain is an *extremely* common problem and one that is often very difficult to treat. The pain is very frustrating to the patient, who has to live with it day in and day out, and very frustrating to the Health Care Professional (HCP), who has to treat it. This is especially true for the HCP who typically has not had any training in any of the so-called complementary or alternative methods of treatment, such as manipulation techniques or acupuncture. Although my health care professional colleagues are sincere in their desire to help their patients, chronic medical low back pain is a very tough problem and many HCPs just don't know what to do about the condition.

When I first started to practice medicine in 1968, I would cringe when people with chronic, medical low back pain walked into my office. I cringed because I felt so frustrated. I wanted so much to be able to help them. I knew that they weren't lying to me about their pain and that they really wanted to get better. However, I felt powerless to help them with the limited number of tools that I had at my disposal. At that time in my professional life, I knew nothing about complementary medicine. I had only two options from which to choose: drugs or physical therapy. However, I hated having to resort to repeated refills of prescription muscle relaxants and painkillers. That frustration led me to look elsewhere for other tools to put into my toolbox of treatment options.

As a western-trained M.D., I have found that the skills that I developed in manual medicine (manipulation) and acupuncture are extremely valuable assets to me in the treatment of chronic medical lower back pain. Talking with my patients, I discovered *many* of my patients with chronic low back pain had *already* been treated by other HCPs with spinal manipulation and acupuncture. Yet they *still* had low back pain. Now, I am not so egotistical to think that I am so much better at manipulation or acupuncture than the many thousands of very highly qualified HCPs out there. So, what was I doing that was making such a difference in the results? That's what this book is about.

Many of my patients ask me if there's anything they can do to help themselves. They are very eager to be part of the solution. They want to do anything and everything, that is safe and reasonable, to get rid of their chronic low back pain. They say to me, "If they can put a man on the moon, then, by God, there ought to be a way to get rid of this damned back pain." Well, if you happen to be one of these people, here's your opportunity.

All of you with chronic medical low back pain who have been frustrated from having tried many different kinds of therapy without good results, and all of my HCP colleagues who have been frustrated from having to treat such a difficult problem, this book is for you. It offers to the patient and to the HCP a simple, safe, and often over-looked approach to solving this dilemma. The information in this book offers you a direction in which to proceed, a simple method to follow and inexpensive tools to use. All you need is an open mind and a willingness to learn. If you take the short time it will require of you to learn this method, most of you will get the relief that you are looking for.

My sincere, best wishes to you in your new adventure.

Harry Oxenhandler, M.D.

ONE

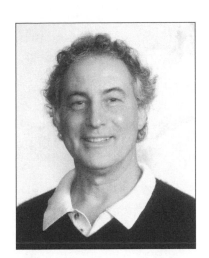

Who is This Guy, Anyway?

When I was age fourteen, I had to undergo some minor surgery. Coming out of the doctor's office after my pre-op examination and walking to the car with my father, I looked up at him and said, "Dad, I want to be a doctor when I grow up." He looked at me with a searching look on his face and said, "You do, huh. Well, I guess we'll just have to wait and see, won't we?"

Having grown up in St. Louis, I did my undergraduate work there at Washington University and started medical school at the University of Missouri in 1962. Between my sophomore and junior years in medical school, I took a year off and went to Germany on a pathology fellowship. I returned and finished medical school in 1967. I did an internship in medicine and surgery at Downstate Medical Center, King's County Hospital, Brooklyn, New York, after which I went into the United States Navy as a Flight Surgeon, where I served for two and a half years.

After the Navy, I joined a small, general practice community clinic in east Redwood City, California. One and a half years later, I left the clinic and began to study acupuncture, because I was beginning to feel frustrated and dissatisfied with my practice. I suppose that throughout my medical training at the university medical center, I was under the impression that when people became sick and went to the doctor, they got better. My experience in general practice quickly taught me differently.

I realized that western medicine was successful at treating many *acute* diseases and successful at treating *surgical* problems. But, western medicine did not have a very high success rate with *chronic* medical diseases, including *many* common, painful conditions, such as headaches, bursitis of the shoulder and hip or back pain, to name a few.

For these problems, the patient had to take prescription medication, which often needed to be regularly refilled. This method was not only quite expensive, but would often result in side effects for the patient. These side effects were sometimes worse than the condition for which the patient took the medication in the first place. Many times, the patient would need another drug to combat the side effects caused by the original medication.

I began to feel as if I were working more for the drug companies than for the patient. So, I started to look around for an "alternative" that would, perhaps, allow me to treat people effectively and, at the same time, more safely. I wasn't abandoning western medicine by any means. I have always felt very proud of much of what western medicine has accomplished. However, I wanted to explore and expand my medical horizons to see what else was out there that worked well. Acupuncture came first into view.

In 1972, there were no acupuncture schools in this country. I learned acupuncture as an apprentice to a woman named Miriam Lee, whom I had heard about from a patient of mine. During the day, Miriam worked at Hewlett-Packard in Palo Alto, California. In the evenings, she had a small acupuncture practice in her home. She had studied acupuncture in her native China and had also learned from her uncle, who was an acupuncturist and a Christian missionary in Taiwan. I studied and practiced with Miriam until 1974.

By 1974, acupuncture was very popular in California. However, there were no laws governing its practice. Acupuncture was essentially an underground activity, well entrenched in San Francisco and Los Angeles. To control the practice of acupuncture, the California Board of Medical Quality Assurance suggested legislation that resulted in acupuncture being legalized and classified as the practice of medicine. As such, only licensed physicians and dentists could practice it. Because Miriam was not a physician, we were asked to stop practicing acupuncture together.

Miriam was told that she could *teach* doctors and dentists how to practice acupuncture, but she could not *practice* it herself. She politely answered with the equivalent of "Thanks, but no thanks." Shortly thereafter, because of a very strong grass roots movement in California, the practice of acupuncture was legalized for qualified non-physicians and, because of her expertise, Miriam was "grand-mothered" in as one of the first licensed acupuncturists in California. She eventually became quite famous as a practitioner, teacher, and author of Chinese medicine. I will always be grateful to Miriam Lee for having taught me acupuncture.

Soon, my practice consisted primarily of Western medicine and acupuncture. In 1977, my family and I moved to Oregon, where I began to build a medical practice. I was invited to become a member of the Acupuncture Committee of the Board of Medical Examiners of the State of Oregon. The job of this committee was to examine prospective candidates for acupuncture licensure and to suggest legislation concerning acupuncture to the Board of Medical Examiners. I was a member of the Acupuncture Committee for approximately five years before resigning due to the increasing demands of my practice.

In the early 1980s, I was involved in a motor vehicle accident and sustained a whiplash injury to my neck. Three months after the accident, I began to have bad headaches. Since I was unable to treat myself with acupuncture for a whiplash injury of the neck, one of my patients suggested that I go to a chiropractor that she knew and liked. I had never been to a chiropractor before and, although I was a little nervous, I finally called the chiropractor's office to set up an appointment. I was so impressed by the positive results of the chiropractic treatment that I asked the chiropractor, Dr. Leonard McBride, D.C., if I could stop by his office from time to time to observe his work with his patients. Dr. McBride and I became good friends and I learned a great deal from him about the benefits of chiropractic manipulation. Unfortunately, a few years later, Dr. McBride became ill and died.

I missed him a great deal, not only because he was my friend, but also because he had helped so many of my patients that I had referred to him. He had such a positive influence on me that, a few years after his death, I decided that I wanted to learn how to do manipulation of the spine and extremities. In 1989, I enrolled in the continuing medical education programs at Michigan State University College of Osteopathic Medicine. Over the next three years, I took over 400 hours of continuing medical education courses in many aspects of manual medicine (manipulation). By the early 1990's my practice consisted of western medicine, Chinese medicine, and manual medicine (manipulation).

In my practice, the majority of patients I currently treat have acute or chronic pain of many types—with the exception of pain caused by malignancy. I also treat lots of people with unusual medical problems (non-painful) that have not responded satisfactorily to western medical therapies. Whereas, many western physicians do not enjoy treating patients with chronic pain because of the frustrations involved in the long-term management of pain medication, I welcome patients with chronic pain because I have a few more tools in my bag.

TWO

The Humpty Dumpty Syndrome

Humpty Dumpty sat on a wall

Humpty Dumpty had a great fall

All the king's horses and all the king's men

Couldn't put Humpty Dumpty together again.

When the idea first occurred to me to write a book on an often overlooked method of diagnosis and treatment of chronic low back pain, I asked myself, "How and why is this book going to be different from the many other books that have already been written on low back pain?" The answer to this question is rather simple. My experience with my own patients has proven to me that the information contained in this book will be very helpful to many, many people with chronic low back pain who have already read other books and have tried many of the other available therapies. This book will offer you valuable and practical insights into the possible causes and possible solutions of your lower back pain. With these new insights, you can begin to take control of and help direct the course of your own journey toward a pain-free lower back.

In my medical practice I treat up to 100 people per week, primarily using western medicine, manipulation, acupuncture, and herbs. Many of these people have chronic low back pain. Many have already been to primary care physicians, orthopedic or neurosurgery specialists, physical medicine specialists, physical therapists, massage therapists, sports trainers, chiropractors, naturopathic physicians, and osteopathic physicians—to "All the king's horses and all the king's men…," —and they still have their chronic low back pain…."Couldn't put Humpty Dumpty together again." I refer to this unfortunate situation as the Humpty Dumpty Syndrome.

I have been a student of the martial arts for five years. When discussing strategy or performing a technique of the martial arts with my teacher and mentor, Grand Master Hyong Kyun Shin, he always emphasizes the following principles: **"SIMPLE, EASY, EFFECTIVE."**

In this book, too, I will emphasize these same principles. I will take you step by step through the necessary "thinking and doing" processes, explaining the method to you in as much "plain English" as possible. There are 140 photos and drawings to help you. You will see how simple the concepts are and how easy they are to understand. Then, after you have read the interesting case histories of real, live patients, you will be convinced of how effective the principles are in maximizing your chances of getting rid of or significantly reducing your chronic low back pain.

Please don't be frightened by the concepts or by the method. You can understand it and you can learn it. When I explain it to my patients in my office, they understand it because it makes sense to them. You will know the "whys and the wherefores." Just take it one step at a time. If I can do it and my patients can do it, you can do it. The method really is simple, easy, and effective. Also, you will not need to come to my office for treatment. You can utilize many of the health care professionals (HCPs) where you live.

THREE

Look Beyond Your Diagnosis

When a patient comes in for a first visit, I always ask for the main complaint. The patient will often answer with a diagnosis instead of what the symptoms are. For example, the patient will say, "I have a bulging disk between L4 and L5. Can you help me?" Another person may answer, "I have degenerative arthritis in my lower back causing pain. Can you help degenerative arthritis?" The patient will frequently bring x-rays or special studies, such as a CAT scan or an MRI scan, which demonstrate such and such a diagnosis, and the patient will ask me if I can treat that diagnosis successfully. This happens quite often for the following reasons:

1. Many of my patients have already been to several other physicians and have been given one or more diagnoses.

2. The patients were told that the diagnosis is the cause of the problem.

3. The patients may have tried many different therapies in the hope of getting better and they want to know immediately if I can successfully treat that particular diagnosis.

In other words, they are sick and tired of chronic back pain and don't want to waste any more of their time and money if I can't successfully treat that particular *diagnosis*. My answer to them is very simple. I do not treat *diagnoses*. I treat patients. Let me give you an example of what I mean.

A patient comes into my office with a five-year history of low back pain. The patient has been examined by the primary care physician and is diagnosed with degenerative disk disease and arthritis of the lumbar spine. For purposes of explanation, let me briefly describe degenerative disk disease. Between each of the vertebrae is a disk, which can be likened to a cushion that acts as a shock absorber between the vertebrae (Fig. 3.1).

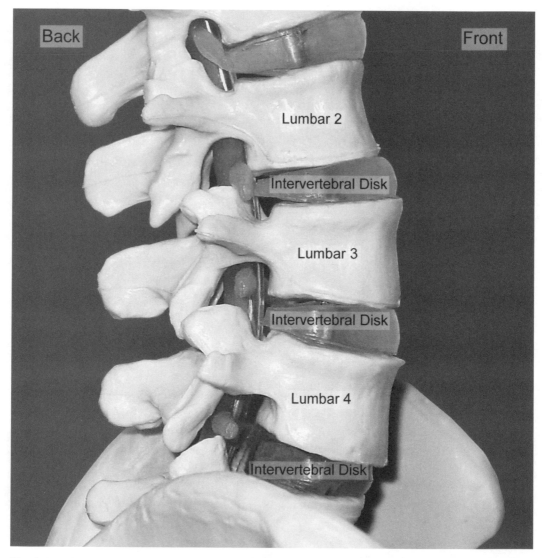

Fig. 3.1 — Side view of a skeleton model showing the vertebrae and intervertebral disks of a normal lumbar spine.

This intervertebral disk is similar to a shoe insert that is filled with gel that you might have seen advertised in magazines or on television. When we walk or run or jump, these disks provide a protective buffer layer between the vertebrae and prevent bone from rubbing against bone. As we grow older, the gel-like substance may harden and become brittle. The disk may also become thinner from the wear and tear of years of weight bearing and, as a result, the space between the vertebrae may become narrower. The disk then provides less cushion effect between the vertebrae. The end result is that weight bearing and other normal activities begin to cause pain. This is degenerative disk disease (Fig. 3.2). Arthritis of the spine, of course, is a condition in which the joints that connect the vertebrae with each other begin to deteriorate. The vertebrae themselves may also begin to show wear and tear. On the x-ray, bony spurs may also be seen on various parts of the vertebrae as an indication of the wear and tear (review Fig. 3.2).

Returning to our example, suppose that the patient's primary complaint is left-sided low back pain, which occasionally goes down into the left leg. Let us also suppose that x-rays have been taken and that they do, indeed, show lumbar degenerative disk disease and arthritis of the lumbar spine. Let's also suppose that an orthopedic surgeon examined the patient and the x-rays and has agreed with the diagnosis. Physical therapy was tried, anti-inflammatory medication was prescribed but both were of little help. The patient was then told that there was nothing more that could be done.

Now, let us also suppose that the patient does not *want* to accept the fact that nothing more can be done and comes into my office with x-rays in hand and says, "I have degenerative disk disease and arthritis in my lumbar spine. Can you help me?" I examine the *patient* and the x-rays and I discover that there are some things that are definitely treatable, so I proceed.

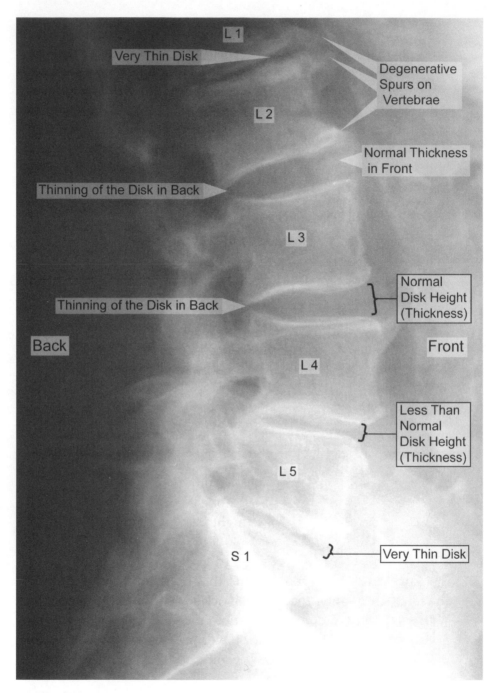

Fig. 3.2 — Side view of an x-ray of the lumbar spine showing thinning of the intervertebral disks (narrower spaces between the vertebrae) and "wear and tear" degeneration of some of the vertebrae (bone spurs).

Let's say that after six or eight treatments, the patient begins to feel significant improvement. After 10 or 12 treatments, the pain is gone and I discharge the patient from my care with instructions to return as needed. If we were to repeat the x-rays when finished with the treatments, would the x-rays have changed? No.

The x-rays would remain the same, showing the same degenerative disk disease and spinal arthritis that had been present before we started treatment. What does all this mean? It means that, yes, the degenerative disk disease and the arthritis in the lumbar spine are definitely there, but they are not the cause of the chronic low back pain. It's as simple as that. Are you beginning to get the picture?

> **A man walks into a doctor's office. He has a carrot sticking in one ear, a banana in the other ear, and a piece of celery sticking out of each nostril. He says to the doctor,**
>
> **"You're my last hope, Doc. What's wrong with me?" The doctor looks at him and says, "It's obvious. You're not eating right!"**

The point of this bit of humor is to illustrate that although it may be "obvious" that the patient is "not eating right," don't you also get the feeling that there just might be something else going on here? Something that is not quite so "obvious" that is *causing* him to not eat right? Similarly, with regard to you and your chronic low back pain, isn't there a possibility that there just might be something else going on in your lower back? Something that's not quite so obvious, something in addition to the diagnosis that you have been given, that's causing your lower back pain? Well, there just might be! In fact, that's what this book is about. So, please read on.

FOUR

What Then is the Problem?

The information that is presented in this book is not new. However, it is not readily available to the average person. This is not because it's "classified" or "restricted" in some way, but because the information has been published in the medical literature, to which the general public does not have easy access. However, in spite of the information having been available, I have found that very few people know about it, including Health Care Professionals (HCPs). I have also found that even if they *do* know about it, many HCPs don't *use* this information even though many of these same HCPs use manipulation techniques in their practice. Whether they don't use the information because these principles were not taught to them or whether it's because they don't believe in them, I don't know. But, I have found the information to be *invaluable* in the treatment of chronic low back pain and I present it to you both—patients and HCPs—in this book.

I obtained the principles, ideas and information in this book from several sources:

1. Articles from the medical literature (Journal of the American Osteopathic Association, Dec., 1979(4):238-50).

2. From my many hours of course work in the continuing medical education seminars offered through Michigan State University College of Osteopathic Medicine.

3. From my thirteen years of personal experience in treating patients with manual medicine (manipulation).

4. From personal communication I have had with Dr. Philip Greenman, D.O., F.A.A.O., Emeritus Professor, Department of Osteopathic Manipulative Medicine, Emeritus Professor, Department of Physical Medicine and Rehabilitation, Michigan State University College of Osteopathic Medicine, East Lansing, Michigan. In my opinion, he is a Grand Master in the art and science of manual medicine. Thank you, Dr. Greenman.

The problem of chronic low back pain and its solution may be so *SIMPLE*, so *EASY*, and so *EFFECTIVE* that many of my patients can't believe it. Patients have often asked me why one of their previous HCPs had not told them about it before. The simple fact of the matter is that **YOUR PELVIS MAY NOT BE LEVEL**. To put it another way, you may have what is called a **"pelvic tilt/short leg syndrome."**

Before we go any further, let me make an important assumption here. I am assuming that most of you have *already* been treated with spinal manipulation by an experienced M.D., chiropractor, osteopath, physical therapist, or naturopath . If this is *not* true, if you have had low back pain for a long time and you have *not* been treated by an HCP that is experienced in spinal manipulation, please find one who is. This simple suggestion, alone, may be the solution to your chronic low back pain problem. If, however, you have already had several sessions of spinal manipulation by an experienced HCP and you still have your back pain, then just sit back and continue reading.

Many of the studies that have been done with regard to the results of treatment of low back pain have suggested that spinal manipulation is most successful in the treatment of *acute* back problems. The studies further reveal that the success rate of manipulation in the treatment of *chronic* low back pain is not very high. *I could not disagree more.* Spinal manipulation, performed by an experienced professional, coupled with attention to the ideas and principles detailed in this book, will yield good results in the treatment of chronic low back pain.

I strongly recommend that you, the patient, along with your HCP, include manipulation techniques as an integral part of your treatment plan. When you do find an HCP who is experienced in manipulation techniques, be sure to present him/her with the ideas contained in this book, because not all HCPs recognize the significance of a pelvic tilt/short leg syndrome or treat it in the same way that I do. I will explain this in more detail a little later in the book. Once, your HCP reads it, (s)he may very likely want to own a copy for future reference.

FIVE

The Failed Lower Back Syndrome

(Humpty Dumpty Syndrome revisited)

The Dirty Half-Dozen

There are several reasons why a person will continue to have chronic low back pain after having seen many health care professionals and having been through many different types of treatment. The reason is that there are several conditions that are often missed or overlooked when a patient is examined. Now, remember, I am *not* talking back problems that are treatable with surgery. We are talking about those people for whom surgery is not the answer: the folks with *medical*, low back pain. These people have been examined and treated by their primary care physicians, physical therapists, chiropractors, osteopaths, physical medicine specialists, orthopedic specialists, massage therapists, sports trainers and many other health care professionals and still have their chronic low back pain. These patients are said to have a "Failed Lower Back Syndrome."

Dr. Greenman often referred to a list of physical findings that may be found in patients with a "Failed Lower Back Syndrome." He called them "the dirty half dozen." *Any one* of the dirty half dozen can cause chronic low back pain. Although it is not necessary to learn all of them in detail, it is important to know that these six conditions exist and to know a little about each one. I will explain, using plain English and photos, what each means. By the time I'm finished, you'll feel comfortable and familiar with them.

One of the "dirty half dozen" causes of chronic low back pain is the *pelvic tilt/short leg syndrome*. I will be spending most of the book on this. However, the other causes of a failed lower back syndrome will be occasionally mentioned. Therefore, if you *know something about each of them,* you can ask your health care professional (HCP) about them. If you have chronic low back pain, *you* may have one or more of them. One more thing before we get started: don't be frightened of these medical terms. I will explain them to you step by step.

The dirty half-dozen are:

1. Non-neutral dysfunction in the lumbar spine and the lower thoracic spine, especially when the vertebra is in a flexed position.

2. Dysfunction of the symphysis pubis.

3. Shear dysfunction of the hip (innominate) bone.

4. Posterior nutation or posterior torsion of the sacrum.

5. Muscle imbalance of the lower extremities and trunk.

6. Pelvic tilt/short leg syndrome.

Remember, don't worry about a few medical terms. By the time I'm finished explaining them to you, you'll say "Oh, that was easy!" Besides, I'll bet many health care professionals don't even know what these terms mean.

As an introduction to the discussion of these several causes of a failed lower back syndrome, a simple anatomy lesson is in order. Please relax. It's just like show and tell. I'll show you a few photos and there will be labels to indicate what the name of each bone is. That's all there is to it. This way, you'll have a much easier time understanding what I'm talking about when I use these terms. They are really very *simple*.

Look at the skeleton of the lumbar spine and pelvis (Fig. 5.1 and Fig. 5.2). Notice the vertebrae of the **lumbar spine** sitting on top of the triangular-shaped **sacrum**. The sacrum is sandwiched between the two large **hip bones**.

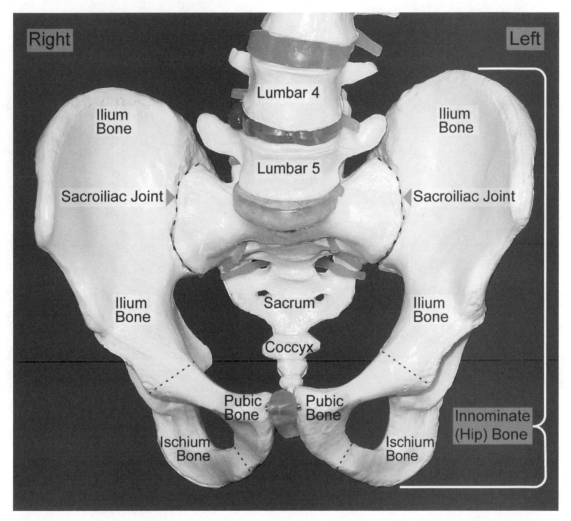

Fig. 5.1 — Front view of the pelvis showing the lower lumbar spine, sacrum and the 3 parts of the hip (innominate) bones.

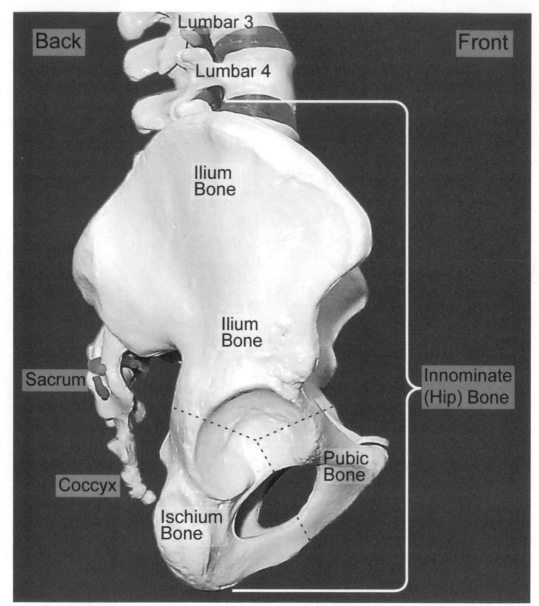

Fig. 5.2 — Side view of the pelvis showing the lumbar spine, sacrum and the same three parts of the hip (innominate) bone.

The large hip bone or **innominate** (pronounced "in-NOM -in-ate") bone is actually three bones that fused together before you were born. The three bones that make up each hip bone are the **ilium** (pronounced "ILL-eee-um"), the **pubic** bone (pronounced "PEW-bick") and the **ischium** (pronounced "ISS-key-um"). The

ilium is the bone you feel when you put your hand on your waist. It is the largest of the three bones. Part of the **ilium** connects with the **sacrum** to form the **sacroiliac** joint (review Fig. 5.1). The **pubic** bone is the bone that you can feel down below where your bladder is, just above where your genitals are located. The **ischium** bone is the bone you "sit" on.

Remember, there are three bones that make up the entire **"hip bone"** or **innominate bone**—the ilium, the ischium and the pubic bone. The photos should make this clear.

Now that we've had a bit of anatomy, let's go back and talk about the "dirty half-dozen" frequent causes of a failed lower back syndrome. In other words, why do people have low back pain even after lots of different kinds of treatment?

1. **Non-neutral dysfunction in the lumbar spine and the lower thoracic spine, especially when the vertebra is in a flexed position.**

Dysfunction means that something isn't working the way it should. When I talk about dysfunction of the spine and pelvis, for example, what I mean to say is that the particular structure in question is not moving freely and easily, that there is restriction of motion in that part of the body. Imagine, for example, you are bending over to lift a relatively heavy object. Your spine is now in a flexed (forward-bent) position, especially your lower back. Suppose then, that you lift the object and discover, too late, that it is far too heavy. You suddenly feel a twinge in your lower back and find that you are unable to straighten up. This is because one (or more) of the vertebrae in your lower back is probably stuck in that flexed (forward-bent) position and "can't" straighten up. More than likely the vertebra is stuck because your back muscles are in spasm and are "holding" that vertebra in a flexed position.

For purposes of illustration, look at what a normal lumbar spine would look like, then look at what a "stuck" lumbar vertebra might look like. Fig. 5.3 shows a side view of your lower lumbar spine.

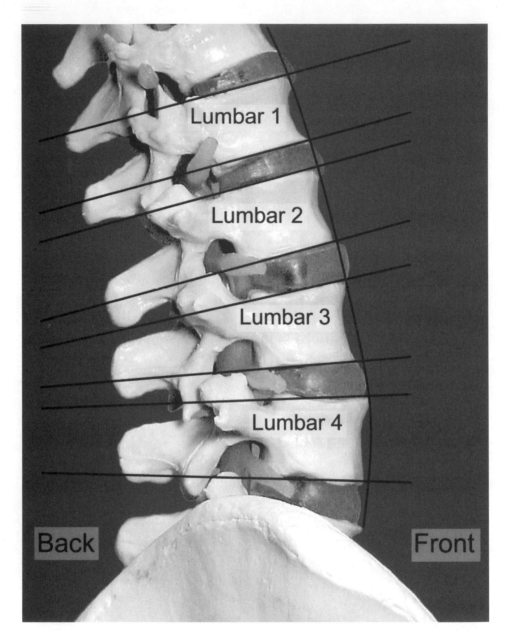

Fig. 5.3 — Side view of the lumbar spine. Notice the gentle, backward curve of each of the vertebrae. This is normal.

Notice the gradual, gentle "backward" bend of each of the vertebrae. The normal, backward curve in the lumbar spine is called "lumbar lordosis." This is how the vertebrae in your lower back normally look.

In Fig. 5.4, notice that two of the vertebrae, **lumbar 3** and, to some extent, **lumbar 2** are "tipped forward" when compared to the others ones above and below them. This is a **flexed, "non-neutral" position of a lumbar vertebra.** If you compare these two vertebrae, lumbar 3 and lumbar 2, with the same vertebrae in Fig. 5.3, you will see the difference. A vertebra "stuck" in the flexed position can cause chronic low back pain.

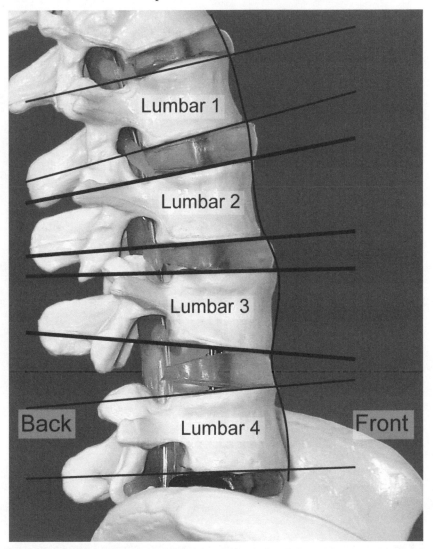

Fig. 5.4 — Side view of the lumbar spine. Notice that lumbar 3 and, to some extent, lumbar 2 vertebrae are "stuck" in a flexed (tipped forward) position and clearly out of alignment with the other lumbar vertebrae (notice darker lines). Compare this photo with Fig. 5.3.

2. Dysfunction of the symphysis pubis.

Look at a photo of the front view of a **pelvic skeleton** (Fig. 5.5). Notice the hip bones, the sacrum "sandwiched" between the two hip bones, and the lumbar spine sitting on top of the sacrum. (Remember that each hip bone is made up of three parts: the ilium, the pubic bone and the ischium that fused together before you were born.) I have marked each of the bones for you in this photo. Note the place where the two pubic bones come together in the midline. This is a joint called the **pubic symphysis.**

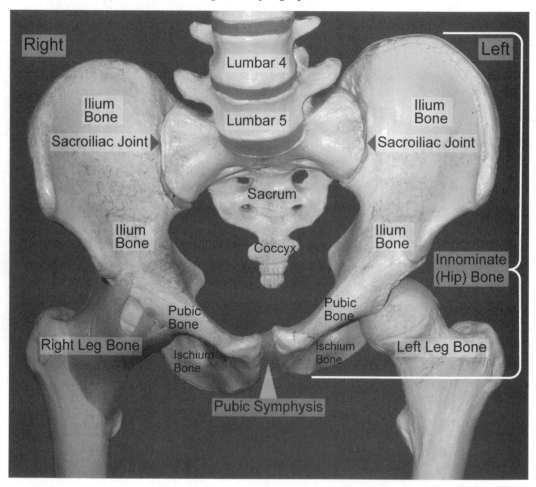

Fig. 5.5 — Front view of the lower lumbar spine and pelvic skeleton with all the bones labeled for easy identification. Notice that the two pubic bones meet in the front of the pelvis in the midline to form the pubic symphysis (joint).

Now look at the *same* structures on an **x-ray of the pelvis** (Fig. 5.5A). Again, see the sacrum sandwiched between the two hip bones. Here also I have marked the ilium bones, the pubic and ischium bones. Notice that the two pubic bones come together at the **pubic symphysis** and meet *evenly* in the midline. This is normal.

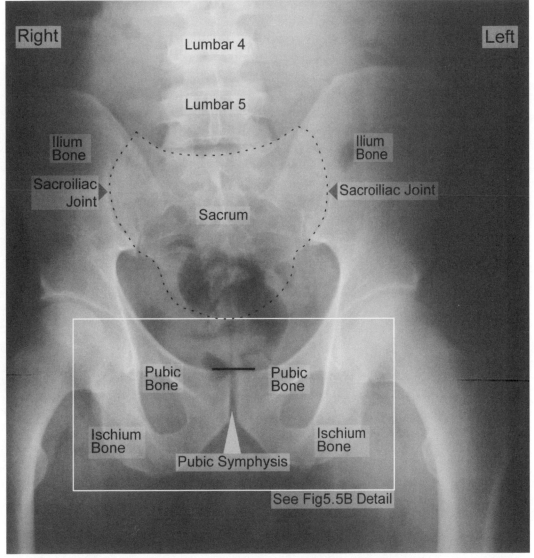

Fig. 5.5A — Front view of an x-ray of the lower lumbar spine and pelvis showing the same bones. Compare Fig. 5.5 with this photo and find the identical structures in each. Notice that the two pubic bones meet evenly in the midline at the pubic symphysis.

So that you can more clearly understand what I'm talking about, look at the next photo (Fig. 5.5.B), which is an enlarged view of the same two pubic bones in Fig. 5.5A. In Fig. 5.5B, one can plainly see how the two pubic bones come together and meet *evenly* in the middle. There are certain conditions, however, in which the two pubic bones do *not* meet evenly in the midline—one of the pubic bones is higher or lower than the other (Fig. 5.6). In this photograph, note that the right pubic bone is lower than the left. When the two pubic bones do *not* meet evenly in the midline, it is called **pubic symphysis dysfunction.**

Now that you have a better idea of what a pubic dysfunction looks like, go back and look again at Fig. 5.5. The skeleton model in this photo also has a **pubic symphysis dysfunction**, because the right pubic bone is lower than the left.

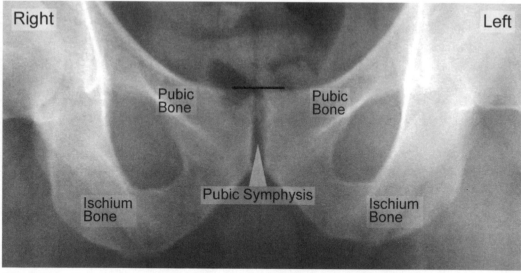

Fig. 5.5B — Enlargement of Fig. 5.5A, showing detail of how the pubic bones meet evenly in the midline at the pubic symphysis.

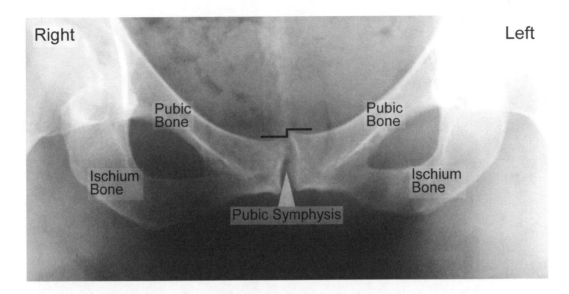

Fig. 5.6 — Enlargement of the pubic bones of another x-ray, showing that the two pubic bones do not meet evenly in the midline. One pubic bone (right) is lower than the other. This is what is meant by a pubic symphysis dysfunction. Now go back and look at Fig. 5.5 again. Is there a pubic dysfunction there, too?

This condition can cause chronic low back pain if not recognized and treated properly. Remember that the diagnosis of pubic dysfunction is made from the physical examination, not from an x-ray. These photos are only to give you a graphic image of what is meant by a pubic symphysis dysfunction.

3. Shear dysfunction of the (hip) innominate bone.

Look at the "normal" pelvic skeleton (Fig. 5.7). Notice that the sacrum sits between the two hip bones and is connected on both sides with the two hip bones at the two sacroiliac joints (dashed lines). Also, note that each leg bone, or femur, connects with the pelvis at the lower end of each hip bone. The reason this is important is explained in the following example.

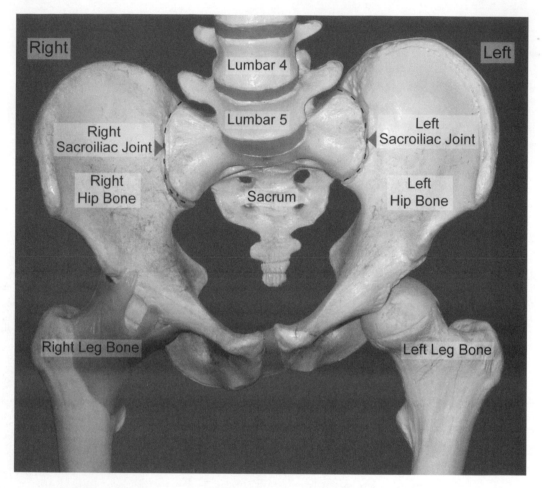

Fig. 5.7 — Normal pelvic skeleton. The sacrum is joined on both sides to the hip bones at the sacroiliac joints (dashed lines). Notice that the leg bones connect with the lower end of the hip bones.

Suppose you are driving down the street and the car in front of you stops suddenly. You jam on the brakes but you still crash into the back of the vehicle in front of you with *your foot still on the brake pedal.* The force from the crash with your foot on the brake is transmitted up your leg to the hip (innominate) bone and causes the entire hip bone, on that side, to shear (move) upward. The upward movement of the hip bone takes place *along the sacroiliac joint and pubic sympysis.* The hip bone can get stuck in this upward position and cause chronic lower back pain (Fig. 5.8). This is what is meant by **shear dysfunction of the hip (innominate) bone.** The same thing can also happen from stepping off a curb you did not see and feeling a jolt in your hip. It can also happen if you repeatedly step down out of a truck and land on the same foot and leg. It may also often occur after a fall in which the person lands on his/her buttocks. As with dysfunction of the pubic symphysis, the diagnosis of an innominate shear is made from physical examination. These photos are simply to give you a graphic image of what a shear dysfunction might look like.

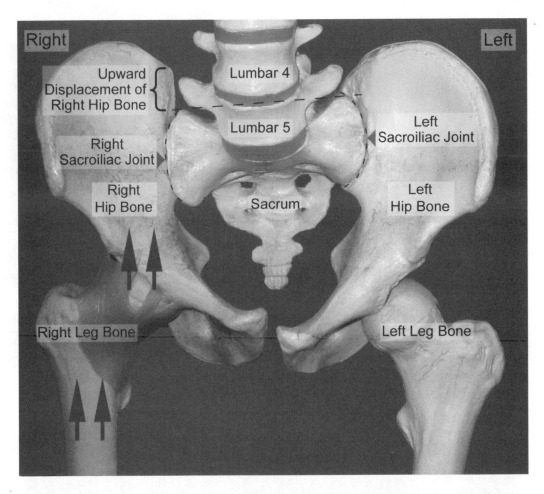

Fig. 5.8 — Arrows show the direction of force transmitted up the right leg bone to the hip bone causing the entire right hip bone to "shear" (move) upward along the right sacro-iliac joint (dashed line). Notice how the entire right hip bone is displaced upward when compared with the left.

4. **Posterior (backward) nutation or posterior torsion of the sacrum.**

    Posterior means "backward," **nutation** means "tipped" and **torsion** means "twisted."

    Looking at the front view of a pelvic skeleton, one can see the familiar, triangle-shaped sacrum in between the two hip (innominate) bones (Fig. 5.9). The place where the sacrum joins with the hip bone is called the sacroiliac joint. There is both a right and a left sacroiliac joint.

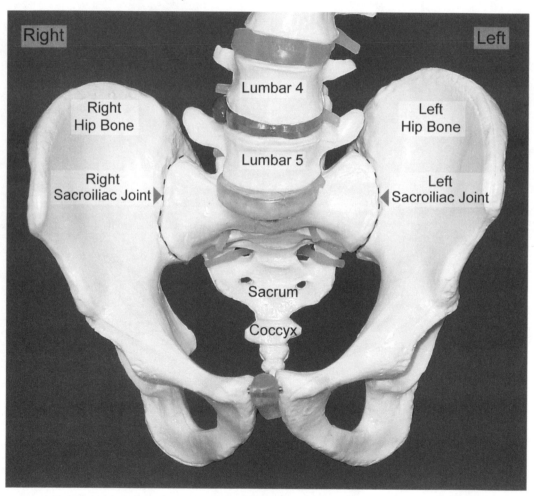

Fig. 5.9 — Focus on the sacrum, which is connected on each side with the hip bones at the sacroiliac joints. The sacrum can move similarly to the way a vertebra does.

The sacrum, by itself, (Fig. 5.10) is actually five vertebrae that have fused together to form one larger, triangle-shaped bone. The sacrum has the ability to move in several directions when you walk, sit and move about. In actuality, even though it is made up of five fused vertebrae, it moves similarly to the way a single vertebra does anywhere else in the lower spine. It can bend forward or "flex." It can bend backwards or "extend." It can also *torsion* or twist forward or backwards, to the right and to the left.

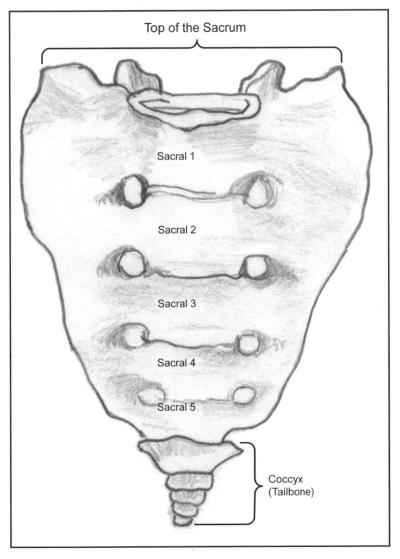

Fig. 5.10 — A front view of a drawing of the sacrum by itself. It is made up of five sacral vertebrae that have fused together to form one, large, triangle-shaped bone.

Fig. 5.11 shows **a top view of the sacrum** as if we were looking down on the sacrum from above. When the sacrum gets stuck in a backward position and/or twists on itself, such as may happen with over exertion or by lifting something too heavy, this can result in a **posterior nutation** or a **posterior torsion.** A posterior nutation or a posterior torsion can cause chronic low back pain. Fig. 5.12 illustrates what a **posterior torsion** might look like. The diagnosis of a posterior (backward) torsion is made from the physical examination.

5. Muscle imbalance of the lower extremities and trunk.

Without the muscles of the body to act on the skeleton, the skeleton would essentially be just a bag of bones. The muscles attach to the skeleton and cause it to move. Muscles of the extremities and trunk usually work in pairs: there is a muscle or group of muscles, which allows you to move in one direction and another muscle, or group of muscles, which allows you to move in the opposite direction. For example, the muscles that allow you to bend forward, at the waist, are called "flexors" and the ones that allow you to bend backwards are called "extensors." Working in pairs holds true for just about any of the voluntary muscles of the trunk and extremities. In certain situations, however, the flexor and extensor muscle pairs of a specific joint may not exert the same amount of strength or force on the joint in question.

For example, your **iliopsoas** (pronounced "ILL-eee-oh-SO-as") muscle is a muscle in the lower back and pelvis. Its job is to flex the hip joint, allowing you to lift your knee towards your chest. It may be much weaker than your **hamstring** muscle on the back of the thigh, whose job it is to extend or straighten out the hip joint. Because these muscles attach to the pelvis, they can restrict the motion of the pelvis if one muscle is stronger or tighter than the other. This is an example of **muscle imbalance,** which can cause restriction of motion of the pelvis and, as a result, chronic lower back pain.

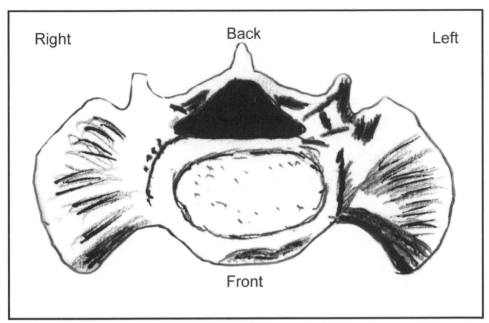

Fig. 5.11 — This is a top view of the sacrum, as if we were looking down on it from above. In this view, the sacrum is in a neutral position.

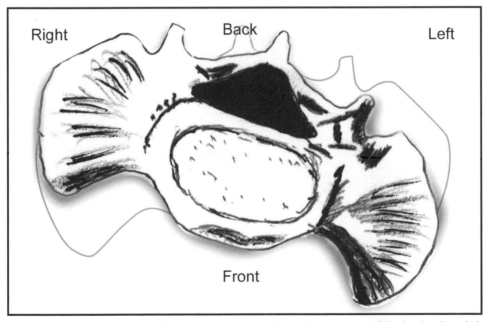

Fig. 5.12 — This top view of the sacrum shows how the sacrum might look when it is "twisted" to the right and "stuck" in a backward position. This is called a backward torsion.

Unless this muscle imbalance is corrected, the back pain will continue. At best, any relief obtained by manipulation will be short-lived. However, through the use of specific, muscle-balancing exercises designed to stretch and/or strengthen these individual muscles or muscle groups, the balance in the amount of force that each muscle group exerts on the specific joint can be restored. In this way, there will no longer be any restriction of motion in that joint and the back pain may disappear. Muscle-balancing techniques can be very useful in the treatment of chronic lower back pain.

Summary

- This chapter outlines five of the six physical findings that are often present and overlooked in people who continue to have chronic low back pain after having been treated by many different health care professionals.

- They are presented because each may be occasionally mentioned later in the book. Don't focus too much on them. Just know that they exist and a little about each one.

- The sixth physical finding often present and overlooked in people with chronic low back pain is the **pelvic tilt/short leg syndrome.**

- The diagnosis and treatment of **pelvic tilt/short leg syndrome** is the central theme of this book and will be discussed in detail throughout the remainder of the book.

SIX

Pelvic Tilt/Short Leg Syndrome

A pelvic tilt/short leg syndrome is a condition in which one side of the pelvis (right or left) is lower than the opposite side. Also, one leg *may or may not be* shorter than the other leg. Pelvic tilt/short leg syndrome is very common in patients with a failed lower back syndrome. *Nearly 2 out of 3 people running around with chronic, lower back pain have a pelvic tilt/short leg syndrome and don't know it*. Think about this for a minute. Practically 2/3 of the people who are treated for constant or recurrent back pain have a pelvic tilt that is correctable.

This statistic doesn't even take into account the millions of people who have a pelvic tilt but, *as yet*, do not have back pain. In my opinion, the presence of a pelvic tilt/short leg syndrome in a person with *no* lower back pain is a potential "bad back waiting to happen." In my practice, I often find a tilted pelvis in people who come in for treatment of problems other than low back pain. I will usually check the lower back, as well. Whenever I discover a pelvic tilt, I always recommend that it be treated appropriately for *prevention* of a future low back problem.

Think about how many people you know with chronic, low back pain. How many co-workers or employees do you know with back pain? How many of them have jobs that require lifting or similar activities that put them at risk for lower back injury? In my opinion, a tilted pelvis, even without back pain, is an unstable condition which makes a person more susceptible to lower back injury.

When the patient comes in for a consultation, I first take a careful history. A typical history from a patient with a pelvic tilt/short leg syndrome is that (s)he was feeling well until one day, after having participated in routine activity, (s)he noticed stiffness and pain in the lower back and, perhaps, some radiating pain into the buttocks, thigh or leg. Often the pain is one-sided and there is usually no associated numbness or weakness present. The patient will go to his/her HCP and, after an examination, be given muscle relaxant and/or anti-inflammatory medication and told to take it easy. If the patient prefers spinal manipulation, (s)he may go to a chiropractor, an osteopath, a naturopath, an M.D. or a physical therapist.

The HCP will treat the acute problem and the patient will feel well for a period of time (depending on the age of the patient, how severe the pelvic tilt is and how flexible the patient is with regard to the musculo-skeletal system). After several weeks or months, another episode of back pain occurs and the patient again goes in for treatment. It may go on like this for months or years, until, one day, the patient becomes aware that he/she has to go in for treatment more and more frequently or even that, perhaps, the treatments are "not working" anymore. Still, another variation is that the back pain which was previously tolerable and did not interfere with the person's daily activities has now bécome intolerable. At this point, the patient and the HCP become frustrated. A number of special studies may be performed, such as an EMG, an MRI scan, a CT scan, or even a myelogram of the lumbar spine.

Consultations may be obtained from either a neurologist, a physiatrist (an M.D. specializing in physical medicine), an orthopedic surgeon or a neurosurgeon. Nobody, however, can find a treatable problem so the patient is told what everyone dreads to hear and what, perhaps, many of you have already heard before: "You're just going to have to learn to live with it." Then, (s)he winds up in my office for a consultation. These are the clues in the history that tip me off to the possibility that he/she may have a pelvic tilt.

Next, I perform a thorough biomechanical or functional examination of the spine and pelvis to determine the exact nature of the problem. By physical examination, I determine which of the thoracic and lumbar vertebrae and sacroiliac joints are working freely and easily and which are not. I pay very special attention to the six, specific causes of a failed lower back syndrome and determine how many of those factors might be present. I then treat whatever problems are present with manual medicine (manipulation).

A very important question to ask at this point would be, "Why would the author of this book want to spend so much time talking about *only one* of the six problems that can cause a failed lower back syndrome?" In other words, why spend so much time on the **pelvic tilt/short leg syndrome** when there are five other causes of chronic lower back pain as well? Here are a few reasons:

1. Whereas the other causes of a failed lower back syndrome (FLBS) must be identified (diagnosed) by a health care professional who is skilled in manipulation, the pelvic tilt/short leg syndrome can be detected by *you* at home with a simple screening test.

2. The presence or absence of pelvic tilt/short leg syndrome can be *confirmed* with a simple x-ray, which you can ask your HCP to do, *even if* the HCP doesn't know anything about manipulation techniques. The other causes of FLBS cannot be confirmed by a simple x-ray. They are confirmed by a physical examination performed by someone skilled in the practice of manual medicine.

3. The five other causes of FLBS, besides pelvic tilt/short leg syndrome, can often be treated with manipulation techniques and/or physical therapy. In my opinion, pelvic tilt/short leg syndrome, confirmed by the proper kind of x-ray, is extremely difficult to successfully treat with *only* manipulation techniques and physical therapy. You will require the use of a heel lift.

You may hear other opinions about pelvic tilt/short leg syndrome from other HCP's. Many health care professionals who are experienced in manipulation techniques either do not know about lift therapy or choose not to use lift therapy to treat pelvic tilt/short leg syndrome. However, I repeat my opinion: pelvic tilt/short leg syndrome is extremely difficult to treat successfully with only manipulation techniques and physical therapy. That is why I want you to know the details of pelvic tilt/short leg syndrome and to completely understand it so you can make an intelligent decision about the kind of treatment you want. The use of a **heel lift** is so *important* in the treatment of chronic low back pain associated with pelvic tilt/short leg syndrome, that it is the central theme of this book.

After you finish reading this book, you will act as a guide to your HCP, taking him/her through the steps to:

- Find out if you have a pelvic tilt.

- Know what to do about it.

I ask you to take a leap of faith that what I am telling you about pelvic tilt works for me and for many of my patients. I wish that all of you could be with me in the office as I see patients. If you could hear the stories that my patients tell me about their back problems, four things would strike you:

1. How *common* the problem of pelvic tilt/short leg syndrome is.

2. How *simple* it is to diagnose.

3. How *easy* it is to correct the underlying problem .

4. How *effective* the treatment is.

To be able to see so many people get better with such a simple (and inexpensive) technique is one of the most gratifying experiences in my practice. Many patients ask me: "Doc, how come nobody told me about this before?" My answer is: "I don't know why nobody ever told you about it before. But, fortunately, you know about it now." Remember, *simple, easy, effective*!

SEVEN

A Screening Examination for the Presence of a Pelvic Tilt/Short Leg Syndrome

The purpose of the examination is to see if you might have a pelvic tilt or a short leg. The person doing the screening places his/her hands on the hip bones of the person being examined and looks to see if the two hip bones are level. Then, the same thing is done with the legs to see if they are the same length. This examination is best done with two people: the person to be examined—the subject—and the person doing the screening exam—the screener. The reason it is best done with two people is because the exam is more accurate when the screener is able to have his/her eyes at the same level as the subject's pelvis. If there is no one else available, then the person can do a self-examination by standing in front of a mirror, although the results will not be as accurate. When you read through the examination procedure below, you will understand more clearly what I mean.

Step #1. The subject should stand barefoot in front of a full-length mirror with feet approximately six inches apart. Having a mirror is not necessary. However, with a mirror, the *subject* can better see what the screener is doing. Have the screener sit on a stool or chair behind the subject. The screener then places each of his/her hands, at waist height, on *top* of each of the subject's hip bones (Fig. 7.1). Making sure that the screener's hands are touching the *top* of the hip *bone* on each side is important. I emphasize *bone* because some of us may have quite a bit of "extra flesh" around the middle. Please be sure to have the screener work the hands down through any "soft tissue" that may be between the hands and the top of the hip bones. The photo of the skeleton of the pelvis has been marked on each side where the hands should be placed (Fig. 7.2).

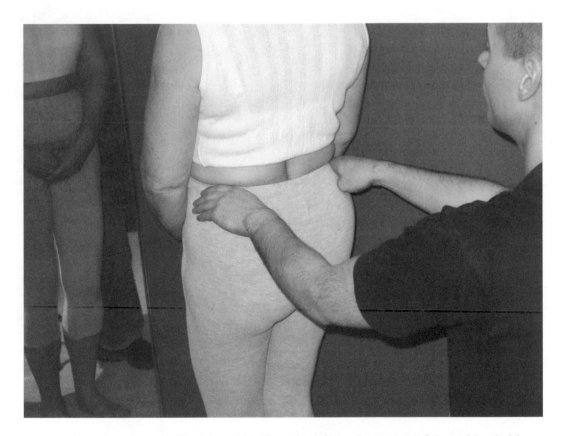

Fig. 7.1 — The examiner has placed his fingers at the waist, on top of the subject's hip bones during the screening examination for pelvic tilt.

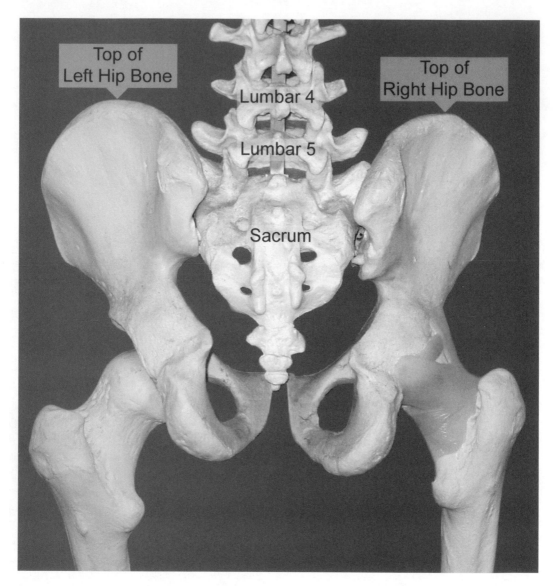

Fig. 7.2 — Back view of a skeleton model showing exactly where the fingers should be placed.

The top of the hip bone is where the subject's waist is, so start there. If there is trouble finding the tops of the hip bones, a simple, helpful maneuver is to ask the subject to **side-bend** to the right and to the left. At the same time, the screener should feel in that general area with the fingers (Fig. 7.3). The tops of the hip bones will become more prominent and easier to find with side-bending. If you are still having difficulty, ask the subject to help you. After all, it's her/his hip bones.

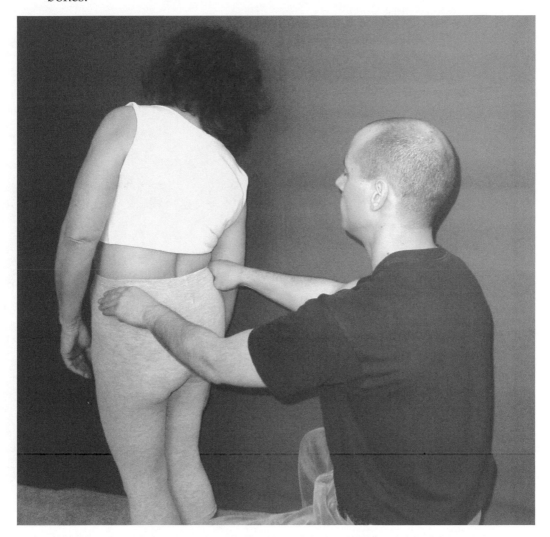

Fig. 7.3 — Shows subject bending side to side, right and left, to make it easy for the screener to feel the tops of the hip bones during screening examination for pelvic tilt.

Step #2. Once the screener is sure that his/her hands are contacting the tops of the hip bones, the screener should lower his/her head so that the eyes are at the *same level* as the hands and look to see if the hands are level with each other or if one hand is higher than the other (Fig. 7.4). If the hands appear level with each other, it means that the pelvis may be level. If, however, if one hand appears even slightly higher than the other, this may mean that the pelvis is not level.

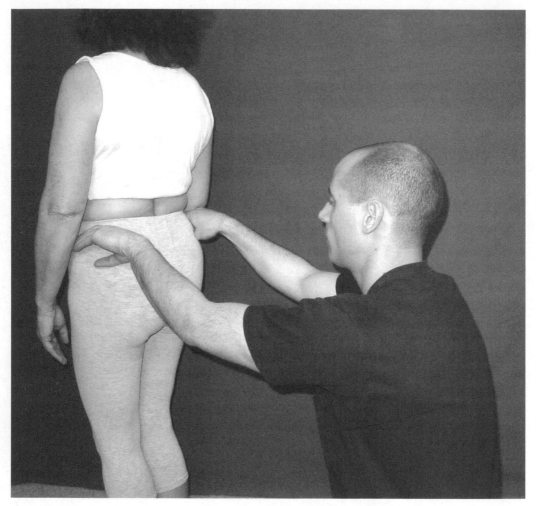

Fig. 7.4 — Shows the examiner with fingers on the tops of the hip bones and eyes at the same level as his hands, checking for levelness of the pelvis.

Step #3. Now compare the length of the leg bones in a similar manner. First, find the tops of the leg bones (femurs) where they connect with the pelvis. For purposes of orientation, look at the photo of the skeleton (Fig. 7.5). The tops of the leg bones are found about 5-8 inches below the tops of the hip bones. Finding the tops of the leg bones is easy. Just have the subject stand in the same position as before, feet six inches apart, with the screener seated in the same way as above. The screener again places the fingers on top of the **hip bones** and asks the subject to do one or both of the following maneuvers:

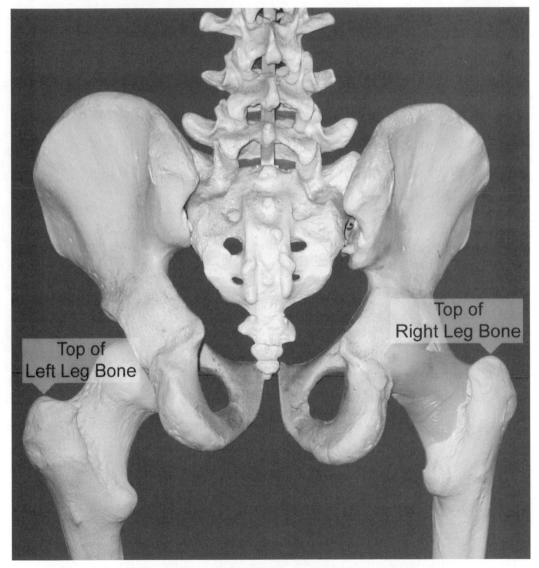

Fig. 7.5 — Back view of the skeleton model with little arrows showing the exact location to place your hands when comparing leg length during the screening examination for a short leg.

1. Slowly move the **hips** from side to side (left to right) (Fig. 7.6).

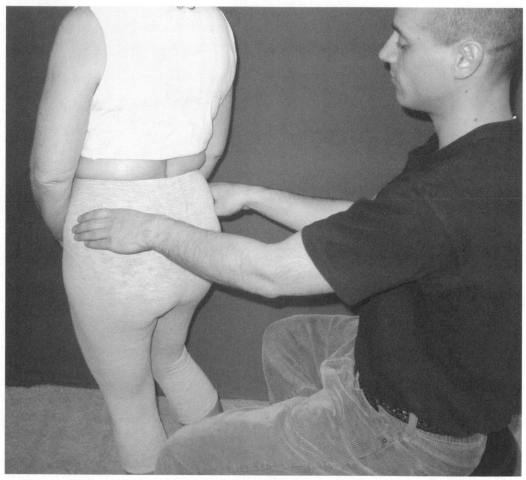

Fig. 7.6 — Subject moves her hips left and right to make it easier for the examiner to feel the tops of the leg bones during the screening examination for short leg.

2. Slowly **side-bend** first to one side, then to the other side (Fig. 7.7).

As the subject is moving his/her hips from side to side or bending side to side, the screener should slowly slide his/her fingers downward from the waist, along the side of the hips. As the subject continues to move the hips left to right or to side-bend left and right, the tops of the leg bones should be felt as prominent

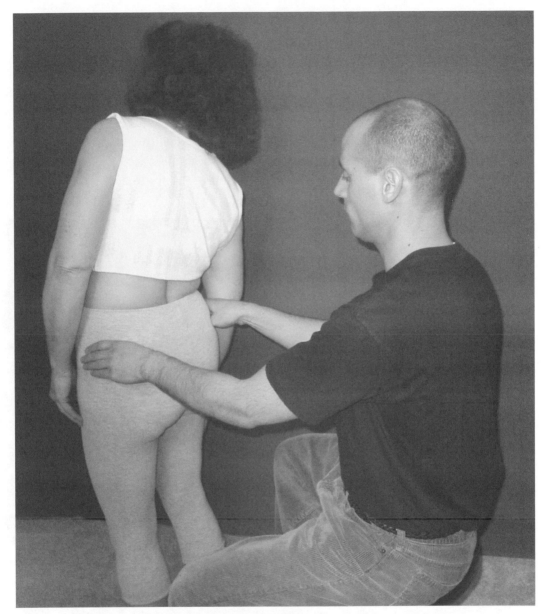

Fig. 7.7 — Subject is side-bending right and left to make it easier for the examiner to find the tops of the leg bones during the screening examination for short leg.

bulges beneath the fingers, about 5-8 inches below where you started. If there is difficulty locating the tops of the leg bones, go back to the tops of the hip bones (waist) and again slowly slide the hands down along the side of the hips as the subject moves the hips or side-bends right and left. Again, Fig. 7.5 shows where the hands should be when the screener has found the right place. The screener can play with it a while until (s)he is sure that the fingers are in the right place. Once the tops of the leg bones have been found, the screener should lower his/her head such that the eyes are at the *same level* as the hands and notice whether or not the hands are level (Fig. 7.8). If the hands are level, this means that the subject's legs are the same length. If the hands are not level, this means that the subject's legs are different in length.

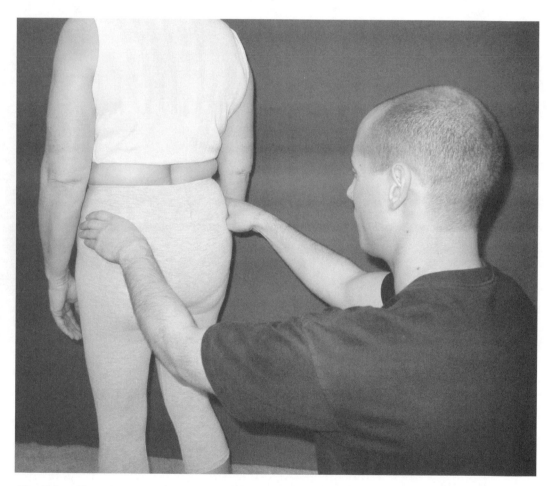

Fig. 7.8 — Examiner with fingers on the tops of the leg bones and eyes at the same level as hands, checking for the presence of a short leg during the screening examination.

To recap, if the screener's hands do not appear level when on top of the subject's hip bones, then one side of the pelvis may be lower and that person may have a pelvic tilt.

If the hands appear unlevel when on top of the leg bones, then one leg is shorter than the other.

If there is any doubt, I would suggest getting a barefoot, UPRIGHT A-P and LATERAL x-ray of the pelvis to determine, for certain, whether or not you have a tilted pelvis. (We'll talk about x-rays later.)

CONGRATULATIONS!!! You have just performed a *simple, easy,* and *effective* screening examination that will take you to the next step in your search for a pain-free lower back.

EIGHT

What To Do Next

Once you have decided that you may have a pelvic tilt/short leg syndrome after performing the screening examination, what next? Do two things:

1. **Tell your health care professional about it.**

    If your HCP doesn't know what the heck you're talking about, don't worry about that right now, because *you* are going to be an expert on pelvic tilt and you will feel perfectly at ease telling your health care professional about it and asking for what you need. But, regardless of whether or not your HCP knows anything about a pelvic tilt, I suggest that you also:

2. **Request that a barefoot, *standing* (upright) x-ray of your pelvis be taken, both front and side view.**

    In my opinion, the *best* way to show that you do have or don't have a pelvic tilt/short leg syndrome is to take a *standing* or UPRIGHT A-P AND LATERAL x-ray (front and side view) of your pelvis. By doing this, you can tell, at once, whether or not the pelvis is tilted and whether or not one leg is shorter than the other. The screening examination will *suggest* whether or not you have a pelvic tilt, but the x-rays will *confirm* it.

    It is important to know that, although pelvic tilt and a short leg are often spoken about together, as if they always occur together, they are actually separate and distinct things. They are not one and the same. They can and do appear independently of each other. I will explain this a little later in more detail. But, for now, just remember that a *standing* x-ray of the pelvis is strongly suggested as the best way to confirm the presence of a pelvic tilt or a short leg.

If after having read the above paragraphs, you are saying to yourself, "I already know that I do (or do not) have a pelvic tilt/short leg syndrome," *but* you have *not* had a *standing* x-ray of your pelvis, then you may be incorrect. An x-ray taken while you are lying down, even if it's an MRI or a CAT scan, won't do the trick. You need a simple, *standing* x-ray of your pelvis, front and side views. Enough said.

NINE

The Standing X-Ray of the Pelvis and The Pelvic Tilt/Short Leg Syndrome

A standing x-ray of the pelvis will tell us, most importantly, whether or not the pelvis is level. It will also give us other information. There are a minimum of two x-rays that should be taken when one gets a standing x-ray of the pelvis: a front view and a side view of the pelvis. For now, we'll consider the front, or A-P, view of the pelvis to see what a pelvic tilt/short leg looks like.

In order to better understand what useful information a standing x-ray of the pelvis can reveal, it will be helpful to review some of the anatomy we learned earlier. First, we'll look at the anatomy of a skeleton model and then, on the same page, we'll look at the *same* anatomy as it appears on the x-ray. It's going to be easy, interesting and informative. The review will come in handy because we will be looking at lots of x-rays.

Fig. 9.1 shows the major areas of interest: the lumbar spine, sitting on top of the sacrum, the sacrum "sandwiched" in between the two hip bones and the two leg bones where they fit into the hip sockets at the lower end of the pelvis. Now look at the photo of the standing x-ray of a pelvis (Fig. 9.2). Here, too, notice the lumbar spine or lumbar vertebrae, the triangular-shaped sacrum, which is "sandwiched" in between the two hip bones, and, lastly, the two leg bones where they attach to the lower part of the pelvis at the hip sockets. There! That was easy!

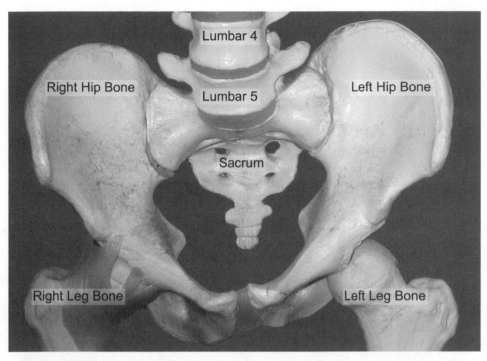

Fig. 9.1 — A front view of the pelvic skeleton showing the familiar bones that you've seen several times before: the lower lumbar spine, the sacrum, the hip bones and the leg bones.

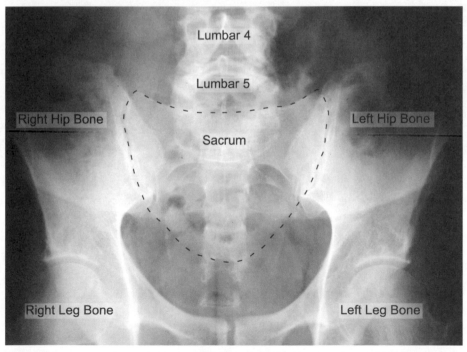

Fig. 9.2 — Front view of a standing x-ray of the pelvis showing the same bones as in the previous photo: the lower lumbar spine, the sacrum (dashed outline), the hip bones and the leg bones.

Now, look at the *very same x-ray* for our next example (Fig. 9.3). This is the same x-ray as in Fig. 9.2, except for one thing: I have drawn one line along the top of the sacrum and another line across the tops of both leg bones. This x-ray is of a normal pelvis and it is normal in this respect: the lines I have drawn along the top of the sacrum and across the tops of the leg bones are *level*. Also, notice that the lower lumbar spine is straight. These are all important factors to remember as we move on to look at another x-ray.

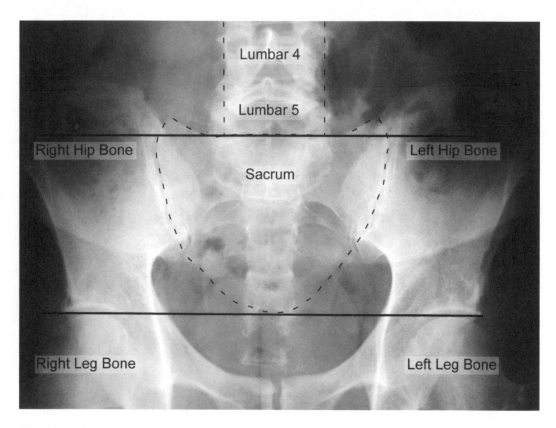

Fig. 9.3 — Same x-ray as the previous photo, showing that the lines drawn along the top of the sacrum and along the tops of the leg bones are both level.

In the next photo of another standing x-ray (Fig. 9.4) you may notice some differences from the previous x-ray. Always look first at the important points of interest: the lumbar spine, the triangular-shaped sacrum sandwiched between the two hip bones and also where the two leg bones attach to the lower part of the hip bones. GOOD!! Is there anything different from the previous x-ray? Let's see.

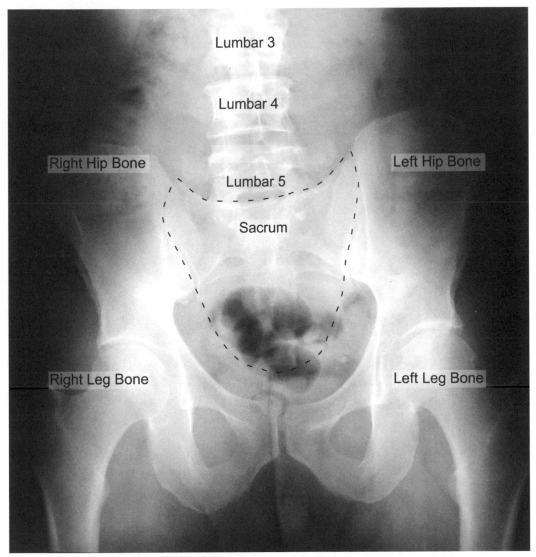

Fig. 9.4 — Shows a standing x-ray of a different pelvis. Notice the same anatomic structures. Do you see anything that looks different from the previous photo?

On this same x-ray, let's draw a line along the top of the sacrum and another line across the top of both leg bones (Fig. 9.5). What do you notice? You will see that the line along the top of the sacrum and the line across the tops of the leg bones are *not level*. The lines

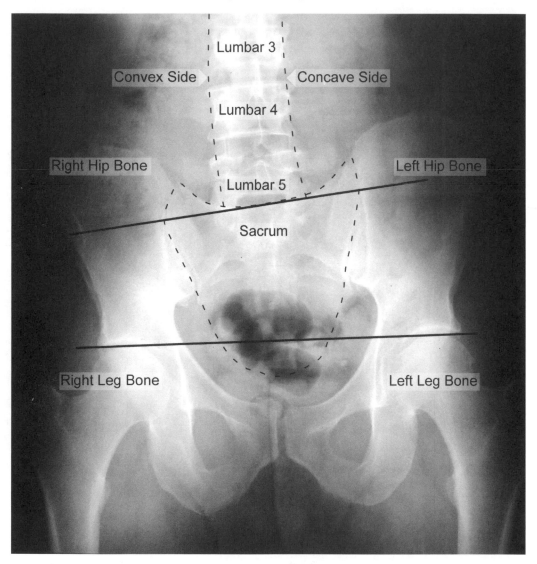

Fig. 9.5 — The same x-ray as in Fig. 9.4 with lines drawn along the sacral base and along the tops of the leg bones, demonstrating a pelvic tilt/short leg syndrome. Right side of pelvis is lower and right leg is shorter. Lumbar curve is convex (bulging) toward the lower (right) side of pelvis.

slope. One side of the pelvis is lower than the other; in this case, the right side. You'll also see that the right leg is slightly shorter than the left. This is what is meant by a pelvic tilt/ short leg syndrome: the pelvis is tilted and one leg is shorter than the other. What an easy concept! Let me say again: in my opinion, *there is really no better substitute for a standing x-ray of the pelvis* to make this diagnosis.

There's something else about this x-ray that is often seen in the x-rays of people with a pelvic tilt/short leg syndrome (Fig. 9.5 again). Namely, there is usually a slight curve in the lower lumbar spine. This curve or "scoliosis" is, often, "bulging" *toward* the *lower* (right) side of the pelvis. In other words, the "convex" part of the curve is almost always on the lower side of the tilted pelvis. In Fig. 9.5, there is, in fact, a slight curve in the lower lumbar spine and the convex side of the curve is, indeed, on the lower (right) side of the pelvis.

Now, let's look at some variations on the pelvic tilt/short leg syndrome. The next photo of a *different* standing x-ray (Fig. 9.6), shows just the opposite. In this example, the line drawn along the top of the sacrum slopes down from right to left. Here, the left side of the pelvis is lower than the right. Also note that the left leg is slightly shorter than the right and, again, that there is a slight curve in the lower lumbar spine which "bulges" toward the *lower* (left) side of the tilted pelvis.

There are other variations that I want to show you, because I want to reemphasize an important point I mentioned briefly in Chapter Eight. So far, we've looked at example x-rays in which, in one case, the right side of the pelvis was lower and the right leg was shorter. Then we looked at another example in which the opposite was true.

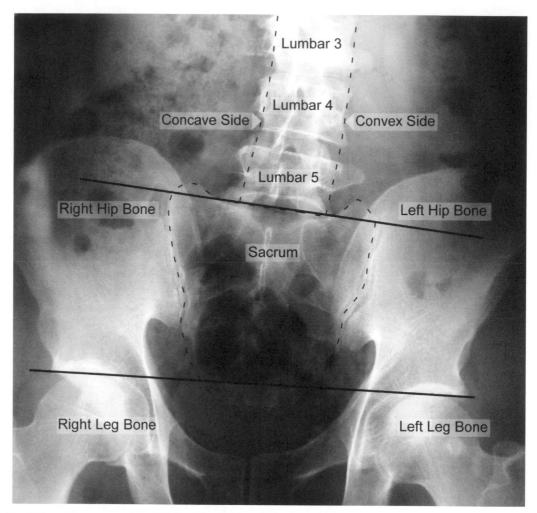

Fig. 9.6 — Shows a pelvic tilt/short leg to the opposite side. The left side of pelvis is lower, the left leg is shorter and the lumbar curve is convex (bulging) toward the lower (left) side of the pelvis.

The other variations that occur with regard to which side of the pelvis is higher or lower and which of the legs is longer or shorter are shown in the simple diagrams below (see Figs. 9.7A-G). Please look at them carefully and then I'll tell you something that will simplify and clarify things about what *is* and what *isn't* important information when it comes to analyzing standing x-rays for pelvic tilt/short leg syndrome.

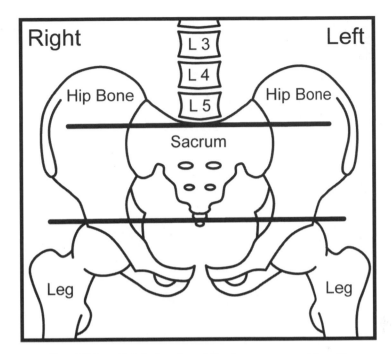

Fig. 9.7A — Pelvis level and the legs are equal length.

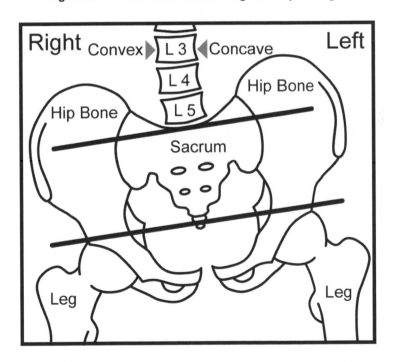

Fig. 9.7B — Pelvis tilted and legs unequal length – pelvis and legs are tilted to the same degree.

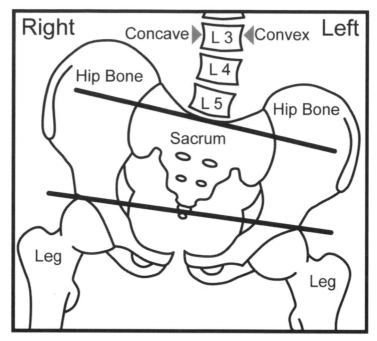

Fig. 9.7C — Pelvis tilted and legs unequal length – pelvis tilted more than legs are tilted.

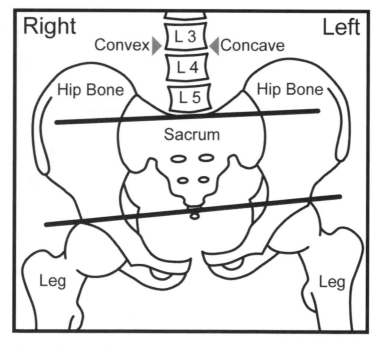

Fig. 9.7D — Pelvis tilted and legs unequal length – pelvis tilted less than legs are tilted.

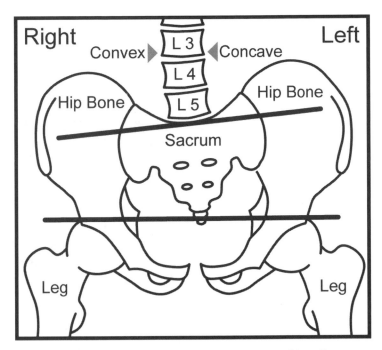

Fig. 9.7E — Pelvis tilted but legs are equal length.

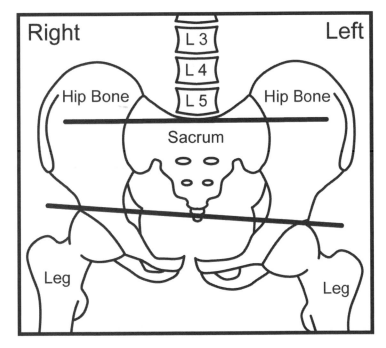

Fig. 9.7F — Pelvis level and (either) leg shorter than the other.

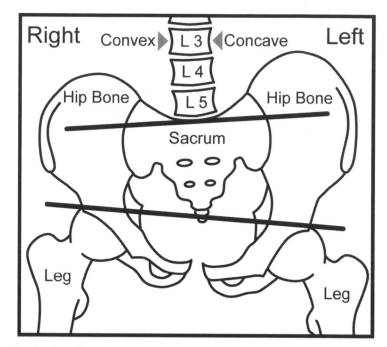

Fig. 9.7G — Pelvis tilted in one direction and legs unequal length, but tilted in opposite direction.

After looking at the above illustrations, you will have noticed that there are *many* possible combinations that can be found with regard to whether or not the sacrum is level and whether or not one leg is shorter than the other. What does all this mean?

It means one thing and one thing, only. *The* most important thing to remember is this: when *analyzing* a standing x-ray and *treating* a pelvic tilt, it does not matter whether the right leg is shorter than the left or whether the left leg is shorter than the right or whether the two legs are of equal length. It only matters whether or not the pelvis is level. In other words, *the most important thing is whether or not the pelvis is level*. Put another way, we only treat a pelvic tilt. We do not treat a short leg.

Please read the above sentence again and memorize it. For years, M.D.s, chiropractors and osteopaths, physical therapists and naturopaths have talked about short legs and pelvic tilts as if they were one and the same thing and debated how to best diagnose and treat them. *What matters most is not leg length; it's whether or not the pelvis is tilted and, if so, how much.*

As you have seen from the above examples, pelvic tilt and a short leg don't necessarily occur together. You can have one without the other. They are not synonymous. Furthermore, I would go so far as to say that the presence of a pelvic tilt and a short leg are often independent of each other.

So why did I give you all of the above information about one leg being shorter or longer than the other and why did I show you how to screen for a short leg if it's not important? I did it because *you need to know about it*. I did it because you may *hear* about it from a health care professional and you may become confused.

You may go to a chiropractor, an osteopath, an M.D., a physical therapist or a naturopath for spinal manipulation and (s)he may tell you that one leg is shorter than the other. You may be put on the examining table and the HCP may ask you to lie on your stomach and then (s)he may put both of your ankle bones or your heels together and, if your ankle bones or heels do not line up evenly with each other, (s)he may tell you that you have a short leg (Fig. 9.8). You also may hear that manipulation or physical therapy or exercises is going to correct the short leg. The HCP may then perform manipulation or physical therapy and, afterwards, (s)he will again put your two inside ankle bones or heels together. If they line up evenly, (s)he may then tell you that the legs are now of equal length and, therefore, that the short leg has been corrected (Fig. 9.9).

You may find this confusing because if you in fact *do* have a short leg, you may well ask how is manipulation going to "lengthen" a short leg? Let me clarify.

There are two different types of "short legs": a **functional** short leg and an **anatomical** short leg. A **functional** short leg is a leg that *appears to be* shorter than the other leg. An **anatomical** short leg is a leg that actually *is* shorter than the other leg. Let me explain further.

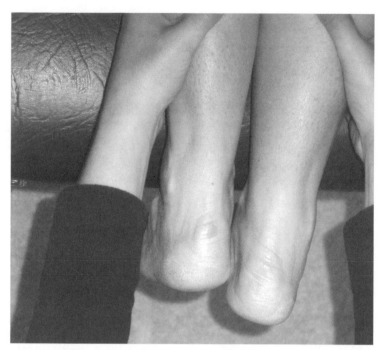

Fig. 9.8 — Shows an example of a functional short leg, which is usually correctable with manipulation techniques. A functional short leg has nothing to do with whether or not your pelvis is tilted.

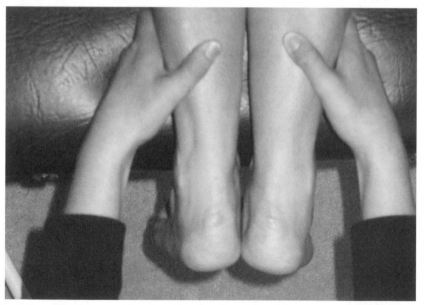

Fig. 9.9 — Shows equal leg length after the patient has been properly treated with manipulation techniques for a functional short leg. A functional short leg has nothing to do with whether or not your pelvis is tilted.

There are a few spinal and pelvic problems (dysfunctions) in which the vertebrae, the sacrum, the hip bones and the muscles which attach to them are out of balance with each other. This is to say that certain muscles will be stronger or tighter than other muscles or that specific vertebrae, the sacrum or the hip bones may be out of alignment. When this happens, the tight muscles may *pull* on the pelvis and leg in such a way as to cause that leg to *appear to be* shorter, relative to the other, when the ankle bones or heels are put together (review Fig. 9.8). This is a **functional** short leg. It's quite similar to the following situation. Try this simple experiment.

Place the palms and fingers of your hands *loosely* together in front of you so that your fingertips line up evenly with each other, your fingers are pointing forward and your thumbs are pointing upward. Next, keeping your palms and fingers loosely together and fingertips lined up evenly with each other, straighten out your arms to their full length in front of you. Finally, keeping your palms and fingers loosely together and your arms straight out in front of you, "shorten" your right arm simply **by pulling your right shoulder backwards a few inches.** You will find that your fingertips no longer line up evenly with each other. By pulling your shoulder backwards, you have "shortened" one arm compared to the other one; at least it appears that way, doesn't it.

This is approximately what happens with a **functional** short leg. It is not *really* a short leg. It just *appears* to be shorter due to the position of the pelvis, sacrum and vertebrae *and* the way the attached muscles are pulling on the leg. With respect to the **functional** short leg, after the proper treatment, the spinal or pelvic problem and the muscle imbalance are corrected. The tight muscles relax and release their "grip" on the sacrum, pelvis and leg and the leg *appears* to "get longer" again when the inside ankle bones or heels are put together and they line up evenly (review Fig. 9.9).

The technique of putting the inside ankle bones or heels together to check for the presence of a **functional** short leg is simply a way of determining if there is muscle imbalance or dysfunction in the spine, pelvis and extremities. It gives the health care professional specific information about what's going on in the spine and pelvis and what (s)he needs to work on. The **functional** short leg *is* "correctable" with manipulation techniques and/or physical therapy. However, the presence of a **functional** short leg has nothing to do with whether or not your pelvis is tilted.

An **anatomical** short leg, on the other hand, is one that a person is either born with or develops during the growth phase of the body. It may also occur as a result of a leg fracture or hip or knee replacement surgery. Most people think that the body is symmetrical, i.e. that body parts on the right and left sides are the same size. This is not true. If you examine your own body closely, you may notice, for example, that one foot, hand, arm or facial profile is different from the other. It is the same with the bones of the body. One can actually be longer or shorter than the other. An **anatomical** short leg can be detected by your screening examination and will show up on a standing x-ray of the pelvis. An **anatomical** short leg *is not* correctable with manipulation techniques or physical therapy and, in most instances, has nothing to do with whether or not your pelvis is tilted.

So, remember these three things:

1. Whether or not you have a **functional** short leg or an **anatomical** short leg doesn't have anything to do with diagnosing or treating a pelvic tilt.

2. *Whether or not your pelvis is tilted* is the most important information we need to know.

3. We *do* treat a significant pelvic tilt. We *don't* treat a short leg.

So, if you have a chronic, lower back problem and if you have already been to *"All the kings horses and all the kings men,"* then its time you tried something different.

You must demand that a barefoot, **STANDING X-RAY** of your pelvis be taken in order to determine whether you do or do not have a pelvic tilt, regardless of what you've been told about your leg length. If you *do* have a pelvic tilt, *then* you have discovered something of *great significance* in your search for relief. In that case, you may need something else in addition to manipulation, physical therapy and exercises in order to get better.

WHEW!! TIME OUT FOR A RECAP

1. Chronic low back pain that has been resistant to the usual medical, chiropractic, osteopathic or physical therapy treatment may be related to the presence of a pelvic tilt.

2. A barefoot, **STANDING** x-ray (front and side view) of the pelvis is the best way to determine the presence or absence of a pelvic tilt.

3. Forget about whether or not one leg is shorter or longer than the other. Just focus on whether or not the pelvis is level, because this is the most important thing.

4. Whenever I mention "short leg" throughout the remainder of this book, I will be referring to an **anatomical** short leg.

5. It *is* your responsibility to assertively request a **STANDING** x-ray of your pelvis in order to determine if you have a pelvic tilt. The name of the x-ray to be taken is an **UPRIGHT A-P AND LATERAL OF THE PELVIS**. I will give you all the necessary details in the next section.

It is *not* your responsibility to know how to analyze the x-ray for the presence or absence of a pelvic tilt, although it's easy enough to do (and I will show you how). It's also *not* your responsibility to know the *details* of how to treat it. It is the job of your HCP and/or the radiologist to know how to analyze the x-ray and it's your HCP's job to know how to treat the pelvic tilt if it's present.

However, please understand this: Analysis of the x-ray and knowing how to treat pelvic tilt are *not* difficult to do. I will be describing *how* in the next sections. I strongly encourage you, the patient, to learn the entire process. It's *easy* stuff and, by the time you are finished with this book, you will be an expert. If, however, you choose not to learn the entire process, I want you to be well enough informed to be a good supervisor that can oversee the initial stages of the process to be sure it's being done correctly. After all, your health care professional may not have heard of pelvic tilt or short leg before, either. When it comes to getting rid of your chronic, lower back pain, "knowledge rules" and you *will* have that knowledge.

TEN

What is Meant by a Significant Pelvic Tilt

For our purposes here a significant pelvic tilt is *that* amount of difference in height between the two sides of the pelvis that is sufficient to interfere with the free and easy motion of the lumbar spine and pelvis and to cause chronic lower back pain. The amount of difference that is considered significant is, in my experience, between four and six millimeters or a little less than 1/4-inch.

If I have a patient with chronic low back pain whose x-ray shows a difference of **five or six millimeters or greater** between the two sides of the pelvis, I will treat that amount of pelvic tilt with a heel lift. If the pelvic tilt is *less than four millimeters*, I will look upon that as, essentially, a level pelvis. If the pelvic tilt is *exactly four mm.*, I will usually treat the patient with manipulation, muscle balancing and/or stretching exercises and observe. If the patient responds satisfactorily to treatment with manipulation and exercises, I will let it go at that. If, however, the patient does not seem to be responding to treatment with manipulation and exercises, I will then treat the 4mm. pelvic tilt with a lift.

Summary

- With a pelvic tilt equal to or greater than 5 or 6mm, treat it with a heel lift.

- Pelvic tilt less than 4mm, the pelvis is essentially level: in other words, don't treat the tilt with a lift.

- Pelvic tilt right at 4mm, I will treat the patient for several weeks with manipulation, stretching exercises and muscle-balancing techniques and observe. If the patient improves and the pain goes away, great. If it doesn't improve after several weeks, I will treat the 4mm. pelvic tilt with a lift in addition to manipulation and exercises.

Now, let's see, in detail, *how* we treat a pelvic tilt.

ELEVEN

Treating a Pelvic Tilt

Pelvic tilt is treated primarily with a heel lift placed inside or on the bottom of the shoe that corresponds to the lower side of the pelvis (Figs. 11.1 & 11.2). If the lower side of the pelvis is the left side, then the lift goes inside the heel portion of the left shoe or on the bottom of the heel of the left shoe. In special circumstances, a portion of the lift may go on the sole of the shoe, as well. This will be explained later in more detail.

Although a heel lift is *necessary* whenever there is significant pelvic tilt, a heel lift, *alone*, is rarely enough to correct chronic low back pain. Often, manipulative care, stretching exercises and sometimes muscle-balancing techniques are necessary to completely correct the problem. However, if you have a significant pelvic tilt and you do not wear a properly applied lift, your chances of getting the long-term relief that you are hoping for will be greatly diminished. *A heel lift is the foundation of treatment of lower back pain where pelvic tilt is present.*

Why are manipulation techniques, stretching exercises and muscle balancing often necessary in addition to wearing a lift? They help the body to adapt to the *change* in the pelvic tilt that is caused by wearing the lift. In other words, the very purpose of wearing a lift is to *level* the pelvis, so that free and easy motion can be restored to the pelvis and lumbar spine.

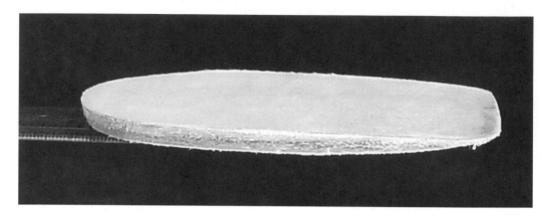

Fig. 11.1 — Shows a typical leather lift that fits inside of the heel portion of the shoe. Notice that it tapers down and will stop at the beginning of the arch.

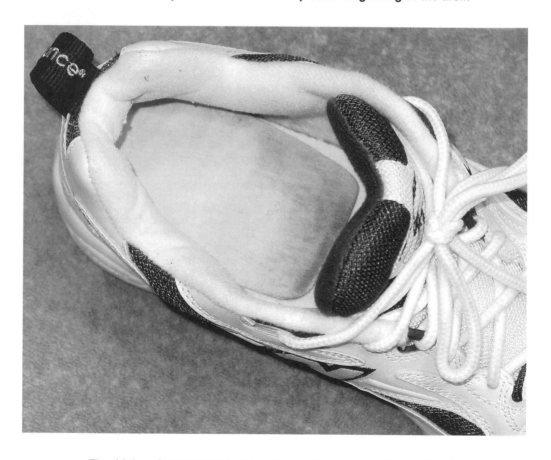

Fig. 11.2 — Shows the lift placed inside the heel portion of the shoe.

Remember that your pelvis has been tilted since you were a child. Because your body *grew* like that, you had *years* to adapt to the tilt of your pelvis. Then one day, you are discovered to have a tilted pelvis and a lift is prescribed. All of a sudden, your pelvis has to adjust to a different angle. Even a 1/4-inch lift is a *big* change for your pelvis to make. This "adjustment" or "adaptation" period takes time. Manipulation techniques, stretching exercises and, if indicated, muscle-balancing will be *very helpful* in correcting any imbalance in the muscles, spine and pelvis, making it easier for your pelvis to adapt to the lift more quickly. Please don't be discouraged by this. Later in the book, you will find several stretching exercises that I give to all of my patients. These have proven to be simple, easy and effective in helping the pelvis to adapt to the lift by improving flexibility.

Treatment of pelvic tilt varies according to the practitioner and most experienced health care professionals (HCP's) will treat pelvic tilt with a heel lift, usually placed inside or on the bottom of the heel section of the shoe. Each HCP who uses heel lifts to treat pelvic tilt has his/her own method of deciding how much lift to start with, how much total lift to give, and how to apply the lift. Understand that there may be some differences among HCP's. The method that I use and will describe has worked for me and for hundreds of my patients.

TWELVE

Once a Lift, Always a Lift

The lift should be worn at all times and forever. Many times I have had a patient come in for treatment months or years after I had prescribed a lift and say, "Hey, Doc, my back felt great until about three months ago." Knowing that I had prescribed a lift, I will ask the patient if (s)he has been wearing it. Often the answer will be "no." The most common excuses are:

1. " I can't find it, but I know it's around the house somewhere."

2. "My back was feeling so well that I didn't think that I needed it any more."

3. "I went to the M.D./chiropractor/osteopath/physical therapist/ naturopath/whatever and was told (for any number of reasons) that I didn't need to wear a lift."

4. "My dog ate it" (most original excuse).

Please wear the lift all the time and wear it forever.

Your lift prescription (how thick the lift is) may need to be re-evaluated and, perhaps, changed later in life. There are a several, very specific reasons for this:

1. Hip replacement surgery.

2. Fracture of the femur or thighbone.

3. Knee replacement surgery.

4. Fracture of the tibia or leg bone.

5. Fracture of the ankle.

6. You begin to wear orthotics or arch supports in your shoes for any reason.

7. Lower back surgery, in which the fifth lumbar vertebra is fused to the sacrum.

If any of these happen to you, please let the HCP who prescribed the lift know about it. (She) may want to repeat your *standing* x-rays because your pelvic tilt may have been significantly changed as a result of any of the above events.

A lift is usually wedge-shaped, thicker at the heel and tapering down to nothing by the time it reaches the arch of the foot (Review Fig. 11.1 and Fig.11.2). The lift should be made of either *hard* leather, like the kind that the soles of shoes are made of, or *hard* rubber. If the lift is made of soft, cushy foam rubber or the like, it will flatten too much under your body weight and not provide enough lift correction.

The lift can usually be made by any shoemaker or leather craftsperson and the good news is it will usually cost under $10.00. If the lift slips around inside of your shoe, just stick a piece of double-sided tape on the bottom of it and it should stay put. You may prefer to have the lift added to the bottom of the heel of your shoe for any of the following reasons, such as:

A. The shoe may not fit properly with the lift inside the shoe. The thickness of the lift may make your foot feel uncomfortable (too tight) inside the shoe.

B. You may want to wear sandals and the lift may feel more comfortable on the bottom of the shoe.

C. The lift inside your shoe may cause you some heel pain.

Wearing the lift inside or outside your shoe is your choice, as long as it's comfortable and you *wear* it. Often, patients will say, "But, I never wear shoes when I'm at home." My answer to that is: "Find a pair of comfortable house shoes or slippers, put your lift in the appropriate shoe and *wear* it!" Of course, if you get up at night to use the toilet, you don't have to wear your lift. You also don't have to wear it when you take a shower. You should, however, slip your shoes and lift on after you get out of the shower and are doing other things in the bathroom like brushing your teeth, etc. Anytime you're going to be on your feet for longer than 5-10 minutes at a time, put on your shoes and lift.

I also suggest to my patients that it's a good idea to *have more than one lift*, especially if you are often wearing different shoes for work or play, casual or dress-up. This way you don't wind up going to a social gathering and discover, after you get there, that your lift is at home in your other shoes and you're going to have to stand around for three hours, in agony, because you forgot to transfer the *#!*#! lift from your other shoes into the ones you are wearing. If that happens, you may be surprised to find you may have a backache that evening or the next day. You probably won't let that happen more than once.

I **STRONGLY** recommend to all of my women patients that they *do not wear "high-heeled" shoes*, especially if they need to wear a lift. The most common complaint that I hear after I recommend "no high heels" is, "But I only wear one-inch heels. Those aren't high heels."

Give me a break! Remember that 6 millimeters (1/4-inch) is a significant pelvic tilt. One-inch heels *do* matter. Further, wearing high-heeled shoes increases the "sway," or arch, in the lower back, that can *interfere* with the *free and easy movement* of the lumbar spine and pelvis, which is what we are trying to promote. High heels can be counter-productive, to say the least.

THIRTEEN

How the Lift Actually Helps

To understand what is happening when the pelvis is tilted and there is a curve in the lower lumbar spine, it is helpful to know something about how the spine and pelvis normally move. Each of the vertebrae of the lumbar spine sits on top of each other and all of them sit on top of the triangular-shaped sacrum. Think of each of the lumbar vertebrae and the sacrum as a series of blocks, sitting on top of one another, with the sacrum as the triangle-shaped **foundation**, or base, of the entire spine. (Figs. 13.1 & 13.2).

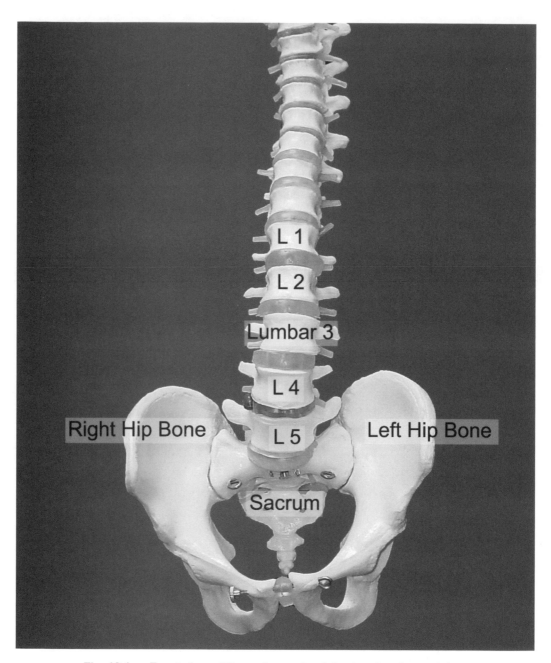

Fig. 13.1 — Front view of the spine and pelvis showing the vertebrae "stacked" on top of each other. The sacrum is the triangular-shaped base or foundation of the spinal column.

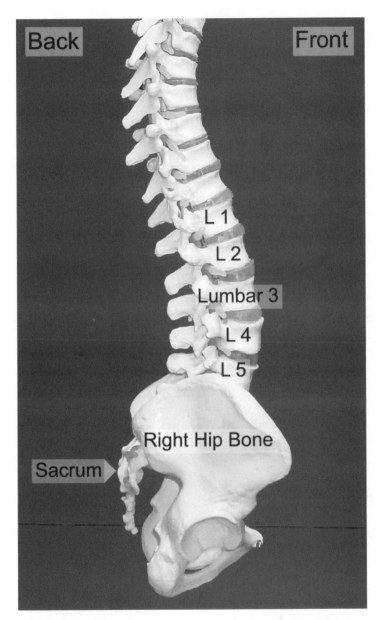

Fig. 13.2 — Side view of spine and pelvis. In the body, the vertebrae and pelvis are all connected with each other by ligaments, tendons and muscles.

Each of the vertebrae and the sacrum and hip bones connect (join) to each other at a **joint**. The joints are bound together and stabilized by ligaments, tendons and muscles. Each of the vertebrae and the sacrum have the ability to bend forward, bend backward, bend leftward, bend rightward, and also have the ability to turn to the right and turn to the left. These movements, of course, occur only when the vertebrae and sacrum are acted upon by the muscles. You understand that if there is no muscle action, there can be no movement. Please look at the x-ray of the front view of the pelvis and lumbar spine (Fig. 13.3). Again, focus attention on the three main points of interest:

1. The lumbar spine.

2. The sacrum, sandwiched between the two hip bones.

3. The tops of the two leg bones, or femurs, where they attach to the lower end of the hipbones.

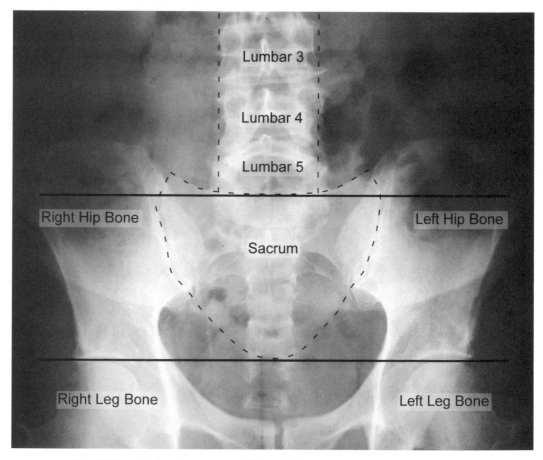

Fig. 13.3 — A standing x-ray of the pelvis, showing that the pelvis is level, the lumbar spine is straight and the legs are equal in length.

Notice in this x-ray (Fig. 13.3) I have drawn a line along the top of the sacrum and across the tops of the leg bones. Note that these lines are level and also note that the lumbar spine is relatively straight. With the sacrum level and the lumbar spine straight, this is the ideal condition for the vertebrae, sacrum and hip bones to have free, easy and equal movement in all directions. Again, when the lumbar spine is straight and the pelvis is level, each of the individual lumbar vertebrae and the sacrum and hip bones can move *freely, easily, and equally* in any direction. This is very important.

In the photo of the next x-ray (Fig. 13.4), pay particular attention, again, to the three main points of interest. Here, the sacrum is tilted down to the right side, the lumbar spine has a slight curve that "bulges" toward the lower (right) side of the pelvis and the right leg is shorter than the left. When the lumbar spine has a curve in it and the sacrum is tilted, it means:

1. That the muscles, tendons, and ligaments that attach on one side of the pelvis and on one side of the lower lumbar vertebra are tight compared to the muscles, tendons, and ligaments on the other side. These tight muscles, tendons and ligaments cause restriction of motion of the lumbar spine, sacrum and pelvis.

2. That if the lumbar vertebrae and pelvis are *already* tilted in one direction to begin with, they are going to be restricted in their ability to move in the opposite direction. When there is restriction of motion, they cannot move freely, easily, and equally in all directions. Pain results when the lumbar vertebrae, sacrum and pelvis try to move against that restriction.

The lift levels the sacrum and removes much of the tension and restriction of motion of the sacrum, hipbones and lumbar spine. Leveling the sacrum also takes the strain off of the tight muscles, tendons and ligaments, and allows the lumbar spine and pelvis to move much more freely, easily, and equally. Where there is free, easy, and equal motion in all directions, there is freedom from pain. This is how the lift helps. What's even better, it works!

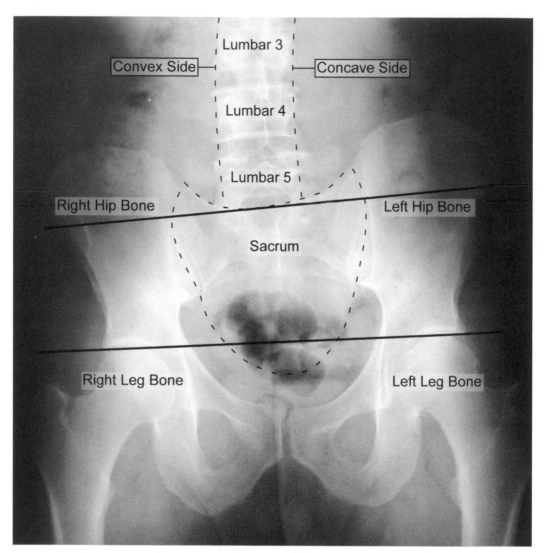

Fig. 13.4 — Another standing x-ray of the pelvis, showing an unlevel pelvis, unequal leg length and a lumbar spine curve that "bulges" toward the lower (right) side of the pelvis.

FOURTEEN

What is the Cause of a Pelvic Tilt

We are not certain what causes a pelvic tilt. One might think that one cause of a pelvic tilt might be that one leg is longer that the other. This would make perfect sense when we look at a photo of an x-ray of the pelvis like the one in Fig. 14.1. Here, the left leg is significantly longer than the right and the pelvis is also tilted in the same direction and, approximately, to the same degree. The left leg is approximately 10mm longer than the right leg and the left side of the pelvis is approximately 10mm higher than the right side of the pelvis. In this case, it seems to make sense.

But what about a scenario like the one presented in Fig. 14.2? In this x-ray, notice that the left side of the pelvis is 9mm higher than the right side but the legs are approximately the same length. Remember our discussion in Chapter Nine (Figs. 9.6A-G) and the several diagrams showing all the possible scenarios with regard to pelvic tilt and leg length? Our theory about leg length discrepancy being the cause of pelvic tilt doesn't hold up in every case, does it? Although a short leg is frequently *associated* with a pelvic tilt, it *may not* necessarily be the *cause* of it, except perhaps in cases where there is a *big* difference in length between the two legs, such as ½-inch or more.

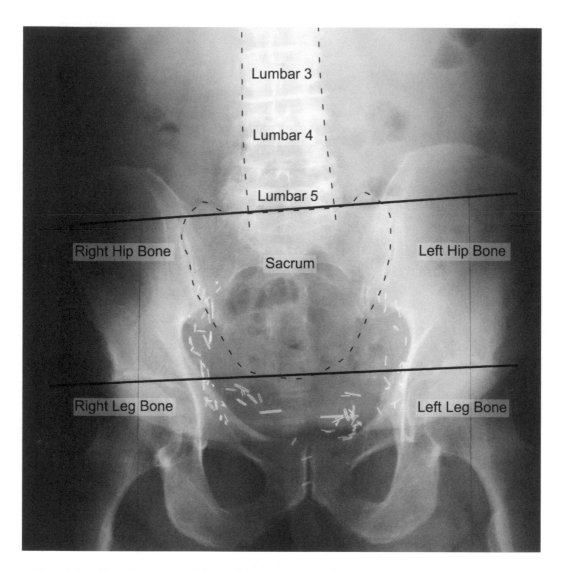

Fig. 14.1 — Standing x-ray of the pelvis shows the left side of the pelvis higher than the right by 10mm an the left leg longer than the right leg by 10mm.

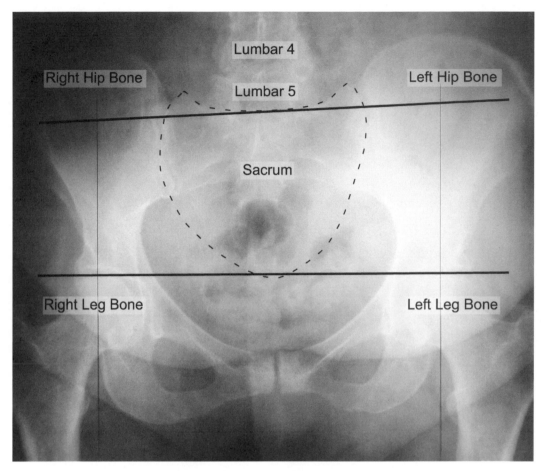

Fig. 14.2 — Another standing pelvic x-ray showing the left side of the pelvis 9mm higher than the right, but the legs are equal in length.

Consider another *possible* cause of pelvic tilt. In Chapter Thirteen, we were saying that each of the vertebrae and the sacrum and hipbones connect to each other by ligaments, tendons, and muscles. With a pelvic tilt and a curve in the lumbar spine, the muscles, tendons, and ligaments on one side may be tighter than on the other side. This imbalance in the amount of force of the various ligaments, tendons, and muscles acting upon the spine and pelvis is a possible contributor to the presence of a pelvic tilt. However, we just don't know for sure which came first: the pelvic tilt and spinal curvature or the tight muscles, ligaments and tendons.

Finally, there may be other factors as well, many of which are not yet very well understood or accepted by most western-trained physicians. One of these factors is the functioning of the cranio-sacral system. This system is a functioning, physiologic system consisting of the brain, the spinal cord, the coverings of the brain and spinal cord, the bones of the skull, the vertebrae and sacrum, and the cerebrospinal fluid. An imbalance in this system may have a very powerful influence on the spine and pelvis and may well cause both a pelvic tilt and spinal curvature.

What's important to remember about pelvic tilt is this: although it would be nice to have a clear-cut, logical understanding of the cause(s) of pelvic tilt, it is not necessary to understand the cause(s) in order to treat it. There are several phenomena in medicine—and in the universe—that we understand only on a superficial level. However, when we go just a little deeper, we discover that we don't *really* understand them at all.

Take electricity, for example. Most people know that electricity is made of electrons. But if we start to go too deep into the origin and nature of the electron, we can argue endlessly as to whether an electron is made of energy or matter. But not having a deep understanding of the *exact* nature of the electron doesn't prevent us from taking advantage of electricity. We just push the switch and the light turns on. Similarly, we don't really have to have a *deep* understanding of the cause(s) of pelvic tilt in order to treat it. When one of my patients asks me what is the cause of pelvic tilt, I will offer the explanations above and then say "It's just the way that your body grew." Then I focus on trying to correct it.

FIFTEEN

Taking the X-Rays
and
Marking the A-P UPRIGHT
X-Ray

The following several chapters are concerned with taking, marking, measuring and analyzing the x-rays and prescribing the lift. These chapters are primarily intended for the health care professional (HCP). However, I strongly encourage *all of you* who have chronic low back pain to continue reading and understand the method. Because if your HCP has had no experience with manipulation techniques, the concept of a tilted pelvis, or the prescription of a lift, then *you*—the patient—will be the one who is better informed. If this is the case, you will need to guide him/her through the method. Better yet, I suggest that you tell your HCP about this book so that (s)he can also learn about pelvic tilt and help you (and many others) to understand and follow this method. Please do not try to do the whole thing by yourself. Ask your HCP for help.

If you choose not to read about the actual method, then please skip ahead to Chapter Twenty-One and finish the book from there. There is valuable information, such as possible side effects of lift therapy, specific stretching exercises and interesting case histories of several of my patients.

First, you will need an UPRIGHT A-P AND A LATERAL X-RAY OF THE PELVIS. These x-rays should include the same bony structures that you have seen in the previous x-rays that we've viewed. These structures include:

1. At least the three lowest lumbar vertebrae (preferable)

2. The entire pelvis (sacrum, coccyx, and innominates)

3. The entire head of each femur (leg bone) and acetabulum (hip socket). If possible, try to include the top two inches of the shaft of the femurs.

Regardless of whether the HCP or a technician takes the x-rays, here are a few, specific technical considerations to remember. They are as follows:

1. The patient must be barefooted.

There must be, at least, one barefooted A-P AND LATERAL UPRIGHT. The A-P is to truly evaluate the levelness of the pelvis: the LATERAL is to evaluate the sacral base angle and the degree of lumbar lordosis. If the patient usually wears orthotics or any shoe inserts, or if the patient is currently wearing a lift previously prescribed by another HCP, an additional UPRIGHT A-P should also be taken with the patient wearing these shoes with the orthotic device(s) or lift in place. Here is why this is done:

Suppose that an A-P UPRIGHT x-ray of the pelvis is taken, with the patient barefoot, and it is found, after measurement of the x-ray, that the pelvis is tilted with right side higher than the left by 9mm (Fig. 15.1). Because the patient has told you that (s)he wears orthotics, the HCP decides to take an additional A-P UPRIGHT OF THE PELVIS. This one, of course, is taken with the patient's shoes on and the orthotics in place. Upon measuring the film, it is discovered that the right side of the pelvis is now 14mm higher than the left (Fig. 15.2).

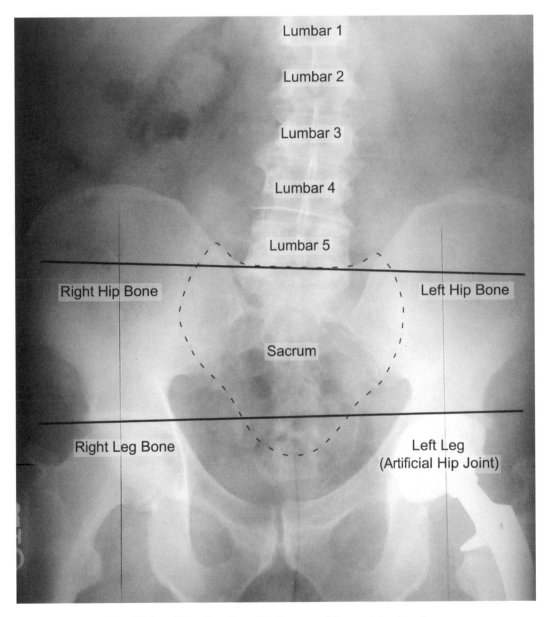

Fig. 15.1 — Standing (barefoot) x-ray of the pelvis showing the right side of the pelvis higher than the left by 9mm.

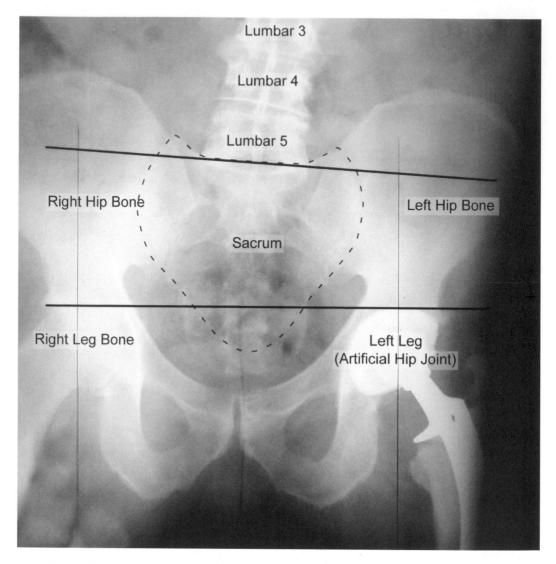

Fig. 15.2 — Standing x-ray of the pelvis (same person) except with shoes on and orthotics in shoes showing the right side of the pelvis is now 14mm higher than the left. The orthotics are not the same thickness and, in this situation, are making the pelvic tilt worse.

What does this tell you? That the orthotics are of different thickness and that when deciding how much of a lift to prescribe, you must take this into account. In this case, the orthotics are *increasing* the pelvic tilt. In other cases, you may find that the orthotics will actually make the tilt less or not change the tilt at all. This must be taken into consideration when prescribing the lift size. Never trust that the orthotics are the same thickness. Always start from scratch in your evaluation of a new patient.

2. **The patient should be *standing up straight* when the x-rays are taken.**

This is important! If a patient having an *acute* episode of low back pain is unable to stand up straight due to muscle spasm and pain, postpone the x-rays until (s)he is able to do so. For obvious reasons, you can't possibly expect the examination to be accurate if the patient is not able to stand straight. Most patients with *chronic* pain who say they "can't" stand up straight, will often put up with the pain long enough to stand up straight for the duration of the x-ray procedure if the importance of the x-rays is explained.

3. **When you send the patient for A-P AND LATERAL UPRIGHT x-rays,** send the following checklist along with the patient to be given to the **x-ray technician** who will actually be taking the x-rays. Better yet, mail a checklist to radiology and talk personally with the technicians and the radiologists to let them know that you will be sending patients for A-P AND LATERAL UPRIGHT films of the pelvis and that you require them to be taken the same way as follows:

   A. An upright bucky that is level with the floor or footrest of the table.

   B. A 14 x 17 film loaded level in bucky.

   C. The patient is standing straight and barefoot with the feet about six inches apart.

   D. There is about 40 inches (1 meter) distance target to film.

   E. The film is vertical and centered at the iliac crest.

   F. The central ray is projected at the center of the film.

G. Remember to tell the x-ray technician what structures you want included in the film (as listed above in this chapter).

H. To reduce mistakes and, therefore, a minimum number of x-rays that have to be repeated, be sure to *tell the patient* what to expect.

Let's go through the actual marking of the films. This is easy. Consider these hints to help you with the process of marking, measuring and analyzing the x-rays in front of you. (I suggest that you read the rest of this chapter, to get an overview, before you actually begin to do any marking of the x-rays. Then come back to the point in this chapter where it tells you to begin to do the marking.)

Step back from the x-rays and just look at them on your viewbox. Look at the A-P view first (Fig. 15.3). Determine if the lumbar spine is straight or if there is a curve or scoliosis present, even a slight amount. If there is a curve present, to which side does it bulge, the right or the left? This may give you a clue to the presence of a pelvic tilt, because the convexity (bulge) of a lumbar curve will usually be on the *lower* side of a tilted pelvis.

Next look at the sacrum. Does it look level or tilted? If it *is* tilted, is it tilted down to the right or down to the left? Then, ask yourself where does the *top* of the sacrum appear to be? Can you find an area on the superior aspect (top) of the sacrum along which you could draw a horizontal line? If so, this may be the sacral base.

The sacral base is the most posterior margin of the top of the body of S1. The sacral base is the most important structure to identify and mark, especially on the A-P UPRIGHT view. It's not that it's so hard to find because it's too small. The problem is that it is sometimes obscured because of the angle at which the x-ray was taken, by degenerative disk disease or arthritic changes at L5-S1 or, sometimes, by contents of the colon. Therefore, some alternatives will be suggested that can be used to determine whether or not the sacrum is level, in case the actual sacral base cannot be precisely identified on the x-ray. You'll see what I mean in just a minute.

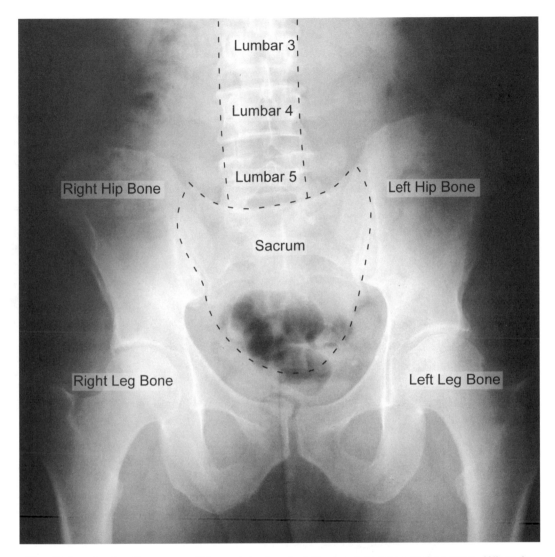

Fig. 15.3 — A standing x-ray of the pelvis. Look at the lumbar spine and sacrum. What do you notice? Is there a pelvic tilt or a lumbar scoliosis (curve)?

Let's identify the sacral base on the UPRIGHT LATERAL (Fig. 15.4). This is simply the most posterior aspect of the body of S1. I have marked it for you on the photo. It's easy to find on the lateral. Now, look at the UPRIGHT A-P view and see if we can locate the sacral base on that view (Fig. 15.4A). It is marked with arrows. In this photo, the sacral base is easily visible on the A-P view.

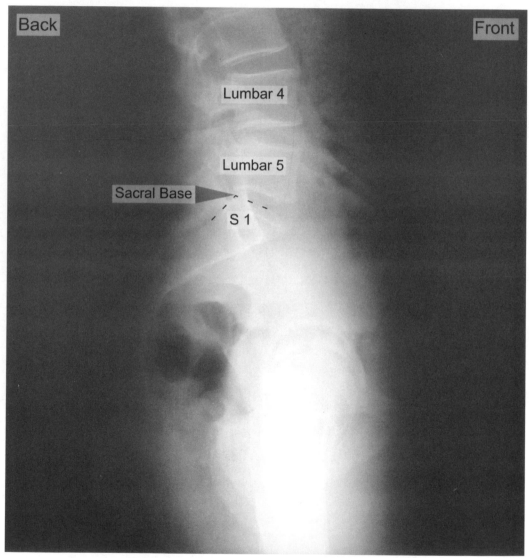

Fig. 15.4 — Shows a standing side view of the pelvis. The most posterior aspect of (back part of) the first sacral vertebra (S1) has been marked. This is the sacral base that we want to identify on the front view.

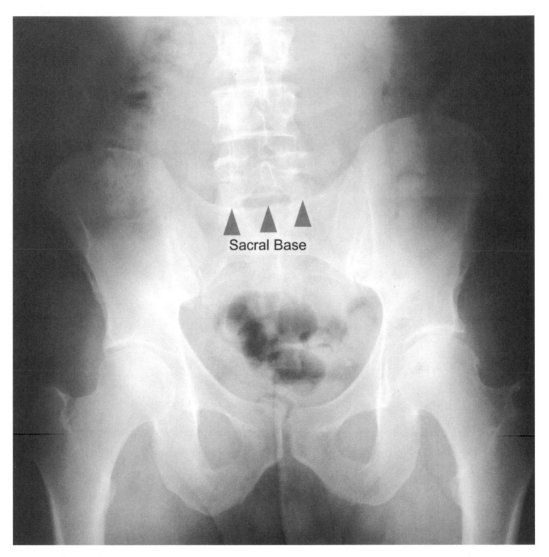

Fig. 15.4A — Arrows point to the sacral base on this standing (upright) front view x-ray of the pelvis.

Then, using a pencil and a "T-square"(Fig. 15.5) or any straight edge and right angle, proceed as follows:

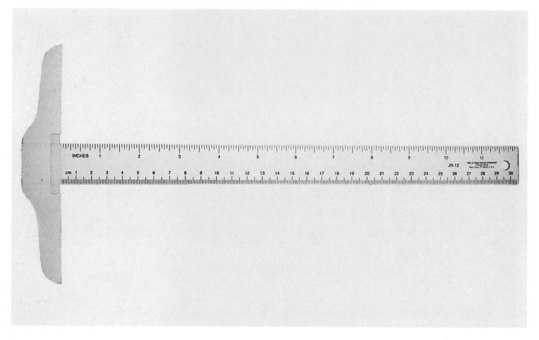

Fig. 15.5 — Shows a "T" square that I use to mark and measure the standing x-rays. Any straight-edge will do if you also have something with which to make a right angle.

1. Draw a horizontal line (AB) along the sacral base and extend it laterally, beyond where the femoral heads (leg bones) attach to the pelvis (Fig. 15.6 and Fig. 15.7).

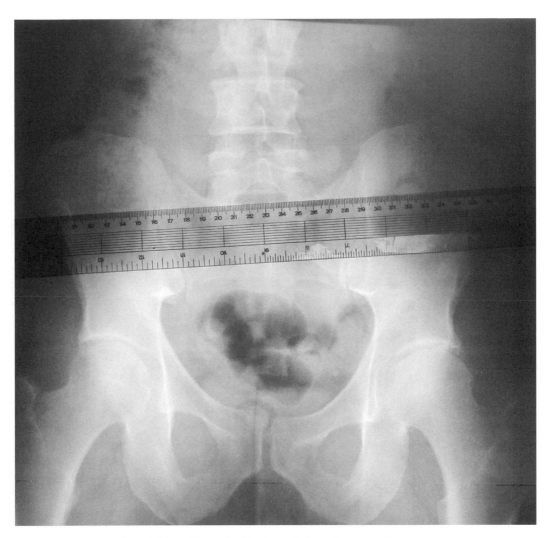

Fig. 15.6 — The ruler is placed along the sacral base.

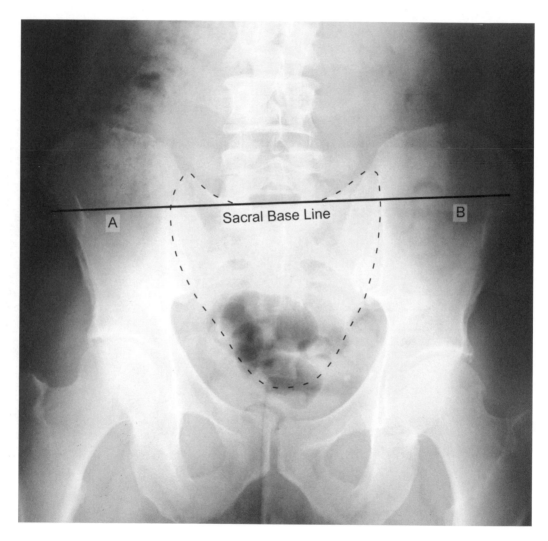

Fig. 15.7 — Shows the line AB drawn along the sacral base and extended laterally beyond where the leg bones attach to the pelvis.

2. Draw two vertical lines (CB and DA) *perpendicular to* the **bottom edge of the x-ray film** that go up and through the *highest point* of *each* femoral head. Extend these lines up toward the top of the x-ray until they meet with and cross the sacral base line (AB) that you drew along the top of the sacrum (Fig. 15.8 and Fig. 15.9).

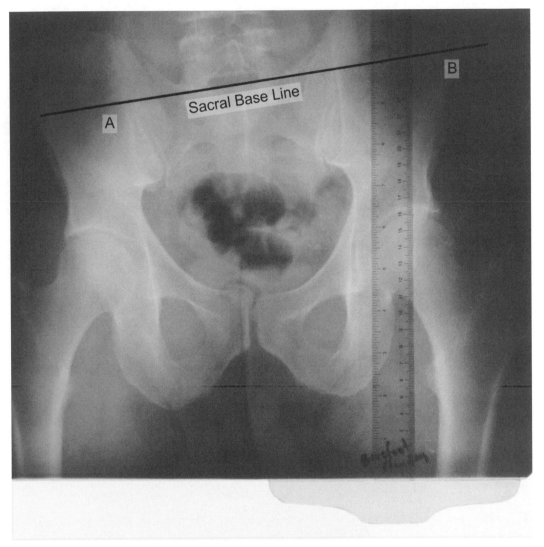

Fig. 15.8 — Use the "T" square to draw the lines CB and DA, which are perpendicular to the bottom of the film; pass through the highest point of the femoral heads and go up beyond line AB toward the iliac crests.

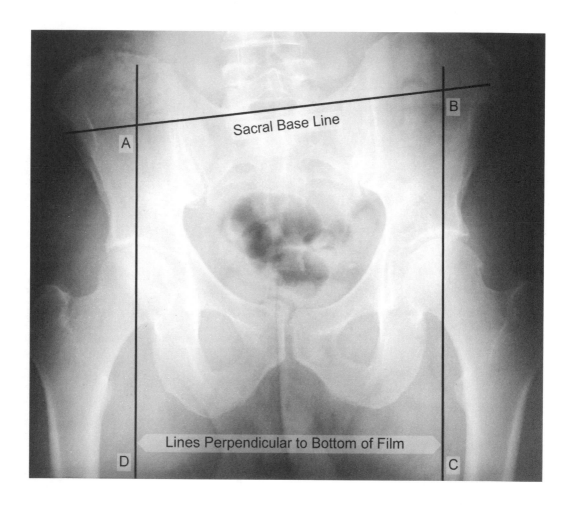

Fig. 15.9 — Shows lines CB and DA, which were drawn perpendicular to the bottom of the film. Lines CB and DA pass through the highest point of each femoral head and extend up toward the iliac crests, crossing the sacral base line AB.

These lines are essential in determining whether or not the sacrum is level. There are two additional lines that are helpful to you in correlating the findings of the screening examination that you did on the patient. These lines are:

3. A horizontal line (EF) that connects the **tops** of the two iliac crests (hip bones) (Fig. 15.10 and Fig. 15.11).

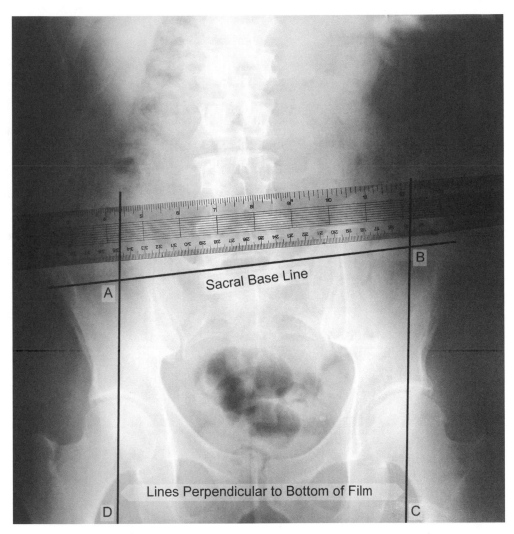

Fig. 15.10 — Place ruler along the tops of the iliac crests and connect them with a line.

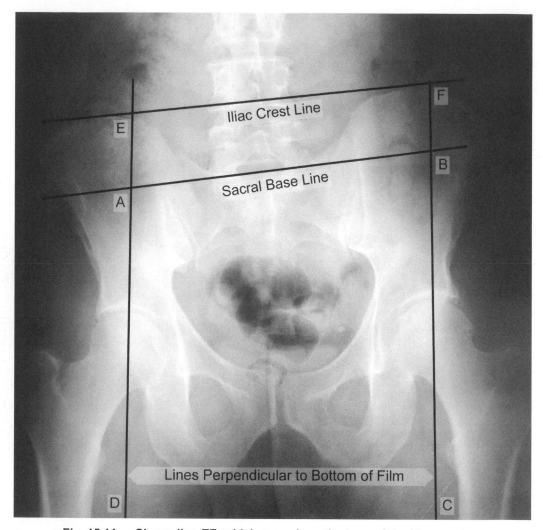

Fig. 15.11 — Shows line EF, which runs along the tops of the iliac crests.

4. A horizontal line (GH) that connects the **tops** of the heads of the femurs (Fig. 15.12 and Fig. 15.13).

Determine if line (EF) connecting the iliac crests and the line (GH) connecting the tops of the leg bones are level. Then remember the results of your screening exam (Chapter Seven) to see how accurate you were in predicting whether or not a pelvic tilt and a short leg were present. Doing this on a regular basis will increase your accuracy.

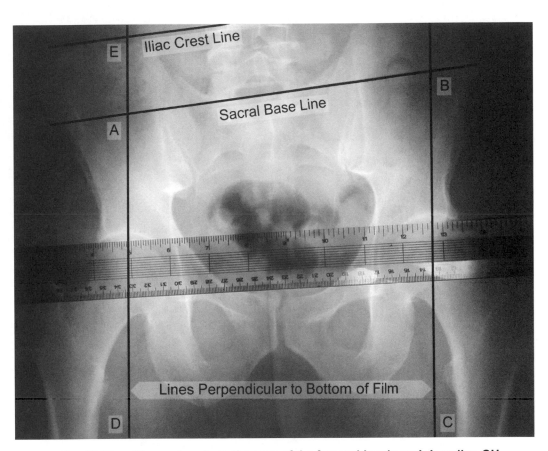

Fig. 15.12 — Place ruler along the tops of the femoral heads and draw line GH.

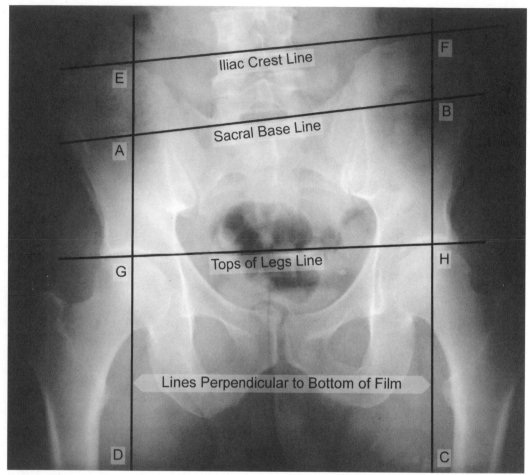

Fig. 15.13 — Line GH runs along the tops of the femoral heads.

Having done all of the above accurately, you will have successfully *marked* the UPRIGHT A-P x-ray. But what do you do if you have an UPRIGHT A-P that looks like the one in Fig. 15.14? In this film, the exact location of the sacral base (the most posterior aspect of the top of the body of S1) is not so easily distinguished. What anatomical structure(s) can we use as landmarks that will give us acceptable accuracy in determining the "levelness" of the pelvis (sacrum) when we can't clearly see the sacral base? There are several, which are listed in order of the most reliable to the least reliable.

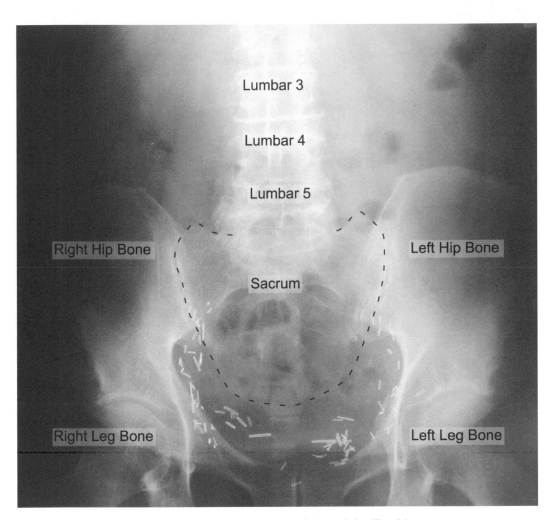

Fig. 15.14 — In some upright x-rays of the pelvis, like this one,
the sacral base is not always clearly identifiable.

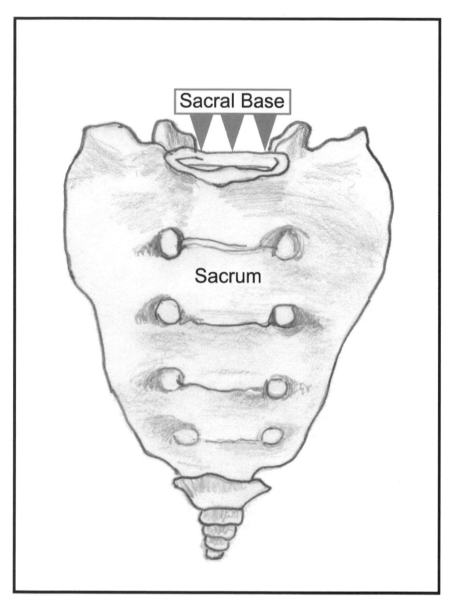

Fig. 15.15 — Front view of drawing of the sacrum showing the sacral base, which is the most posterior aspect of (back part of) the top of S1.

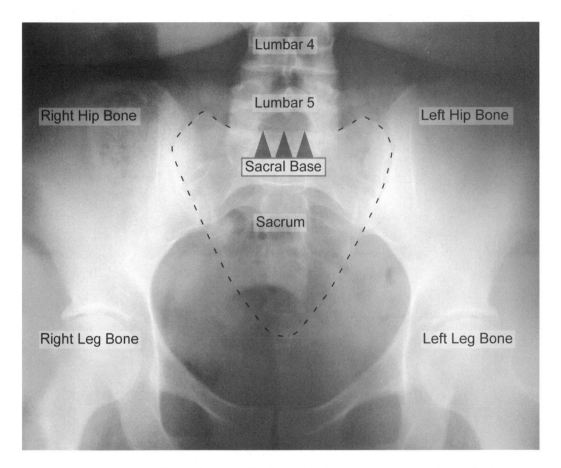

Fig. 15.16 — Standing A-P x-ray of pelvis with the sacral base clearly marked.

1. A **horizontal line** along the **most posterior margin of the top of the body of S1**. This is the **sacral base** as we discussed above (Fig. 15.15 and Fig. 15.16). This should be used whenever it is clearly visible.

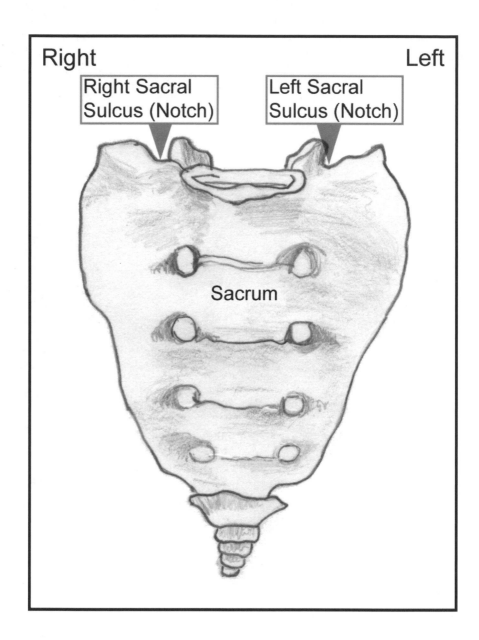

Fig. 15.17 — Drawing of sacrum showing the location of the sacral sulci (notches).

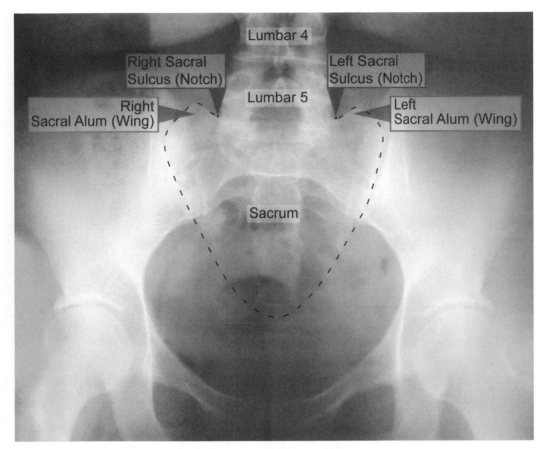

Fig. 15.18 — Upright A-P x-ray of pelvis showing the location of the sacral sulci (notches). The sulci are just medial to (inside of) the sacral ala (wings).

2. A **horizontal line** that connects **equal points on the sacral sulci** *(notches)* located on the superior aspect (top) of each side of the sacrum, just medial to the sacral ala (wings). See Fig. 15.17 and Fig. 15.18. Use these landmarks if the sacral base is not clearly visible, but know that the sacrum must be symmetric for these landmarks to be accurate.

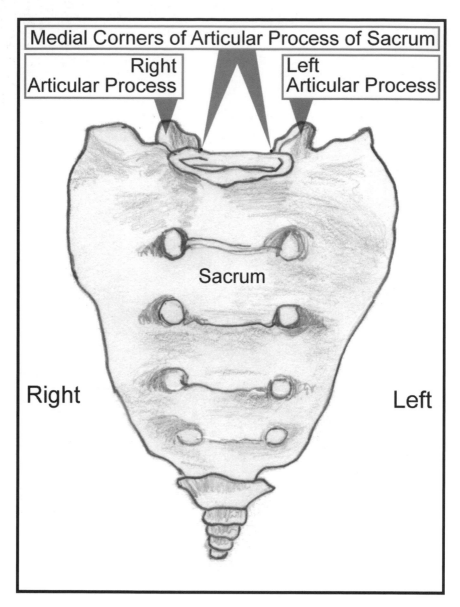

Fig. 15.19 — Sacral drawing identifying the articular processes and the medial corners of the sacral articular processes.

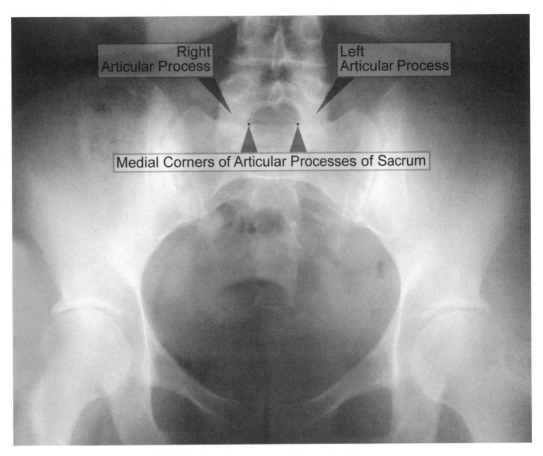

Fig. 15.20 — A-P upright of pelvis locating the articular processes and the medial corners of the sacral articular processes.

3. A **horizontal line** that connects the **medial corner of each of the S1 articular processes**, on each side of the sacrum, where the articular process joins with the sacral body (Fig. 15.19 and Fig. 15.20). Use these landmarks whenever #1. and #2. above are not clearly visible.

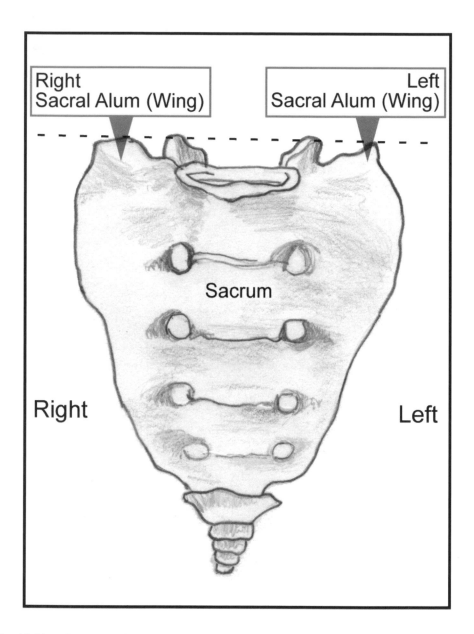

Fig. 15.21 — Drawing of sacrum with sacral ala (wings) marked for easy identification.

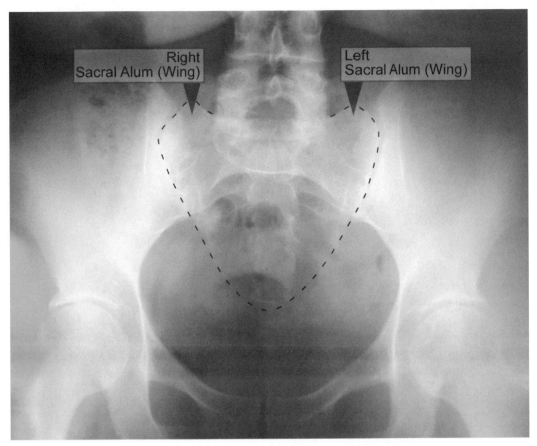

Fig. 15.22 — Sacral ala clearly marked on this upright A-P of the pelvis. Draw a horizontal line across the tops of the two sacral ala.

There are two more alternatives, which I have found satisfactory, but *less reliable* in cases where the above structures are obscured:

    4. A horizontal line connecting the **tops** of the **sacral ala** (Fig. 15.21 and Fig. 15.22).

5. A horizontal line along the **most inferior aspect of the lumbar vertebral body that sits on top of the sacrum** (most often L5) (Fig. 15.23 and Fig. 15.24).

Don't be confused by these alternatives for the sacral base. What you are looking for is this:

A. A reliable **pair** of **corresponding** landmarks on each side of the sacrum that you can connect with a horizontal line.

B. That will, essentially, give you the horizontal plane (levelness) of the sacrum.

C. Follow the order suggested above for greatest reliability.

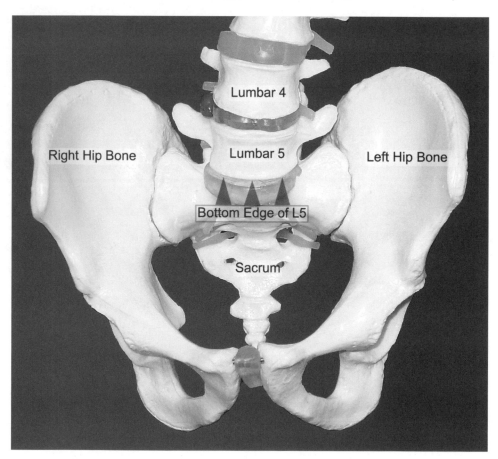

Fig. 15.23 — Skeletal model with the inferior (bottom) edge of L5 identified.

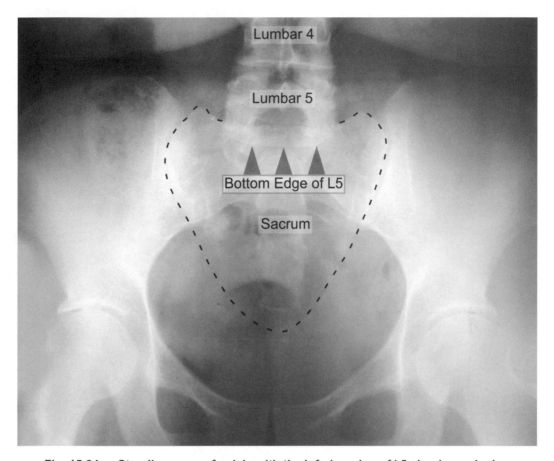

Lumbar 4

Lumbar 5

Bottom Edge of L5

Sacrum

Fig. 15.24 — Standing x-ray of pelvis with the inferior edge of L5 clearly marked.

Much of the time, the sacral base, the sacral sulci (notches) or the medial corners of the sacral articular processes will be visible, making it easy to establish the levelness of the pelvis. Occasionally, you may have to use the sacral ala. On the rare occasion, you may have to use the most inferior aspect of the body of L5.

The landmarks listed above have worked well for me. You should consult with your local radiologists and let them know the kind of information you will be wanting from the requested x-rays. The radiologist should be able to find these radiographic landmarks rather easily and help you identify them on the x-rays. I always read my own films with regard to pelvic tilt. After a short while, you will become good at it.

I'm giving you all the hints that I have learned and discovered over the years that have made it easier for me to evaluate x-rays for the presence of a tilt. Two situations, which occasionally arise are:

- The presence of partial (one-side) or complete (both sides) **sacralization** (Fig. 15.25) of the lowest lumbar vertebra

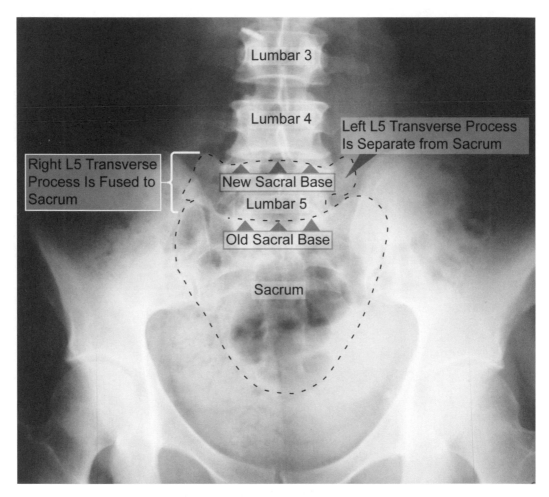

Fig. 15.25 — Upright A-P pelvis showing partial sacralization (right side only) of L5. Therefore, we must use top of L5 as the "new" sacral base.

• Partial **lumbarization** of the first sacral vertebra (Fig. 15.26). The general rule in this situation is this:

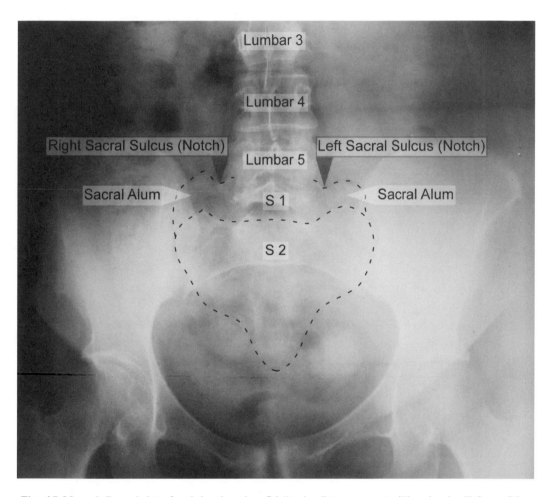

Fig. 15.26 — A-P upright of pelvis showing S1 "trying" to separate ("lumbarize") from S2 but is still fused to the main body of the sacrum, so we use the top of S1 as the sacral base. However, since the sacral base (top of S1) is not clearly visible, we use the sacral sulci (notches), which are clearly visible. We would draw a horizontal line to connect them and use that line as the sacral base.

Whether or not there is complete or partial sacralization/lumbarization, the "sacral base" is considered to be the **most superior aspect** of whatever is partially or completely connected to the sacrum. For example, if L5 is partially (on one side only) attached to the sacrum (sacralized), then the sacral base" is considered to be the most superior aspect of the body of L5. In this case, draw a horizontal line across the most superior aspect of the body of L5 and use it as the "new sacral base." If L5 is completely (on both sides) sacralized or fused to the sacrum, then the same rule applies (use the most superior aspect of the body of L5 as the "new sacral base").

The same thing applies if there has been a surgical fusion of the lumbar spine at L5-S1. Treat it as if L5 were congenitally fused to the sacrum (use the top of the L5 vertebral body as the "new sacral base"). It's really quite simple (review Fig. 15.25).

Where there is partial lumbarization of the first sacral vertebra, the same principle applies. Look for the sacral base, sulci (notches) or medial corners of the S1 articular processes to determine the levelness of the sacrum (review Fig. 15.26).

Another hint that will occasionally help you avoid repeating a series of x-rays is this: For patients who are constipated, a laxative should be prescribed before the x-rays are taken. Patients who are constipated may have gas and fecal material in the colon that can easily obscure the bony landmarks you will rely on to accurately mark and measure the x-rays. If the patient's history or physical examination (palpation of the abdomen) suggests it, a mild laxative may save you and the patient the inconvenience of repeating x-rays.

Summary

- Follow the simple suggestions listed in the first few pages of this chapter with regard to how to have the x-ray taken.

- Identify and mark the sacral base or the next best alternative. The order of most reliable alternative to least reliable is:

- A line along the sacral base.

- A line connecting the sacral sulci (notches).

- A line connecting the medial corners of the sacral articular processes where they connect with the body of the sacrum.

- A line connecting the tops of the sacral ala.

- A line along the inferior edge of the lowest lumbar vertebrae (usually L5).

- Lumbarization and sacralization are special circumstances which occur not infrequently. Follow the guidelines in the chapter.

SIXTEEN

Measuring the
A-P UPRIGHT X-Ray

Now that the A-P view has been marked, it is ready to be measured. This, too, is very simple. You already know what tools you will need to measure the x-rays, so let's begin.

Although I use the metric side of the straight edge, the inch side works as well. Just be consistent. Put the x-ray on your viewbox. To determine whether or not there is a pelvic tilt, simply measure the length of both of the lines, CB and DA, that you have already drawn from the bottom of the film (Fig. 16.1 and Fig. 16.2). Compare the length of each line. Any difference between the length of these two lines represents the amount of pelvic tilt. If the lengths of the lines are within 3-4 millimeters of each other, there is no significant tilt present (see Chapter Ten).

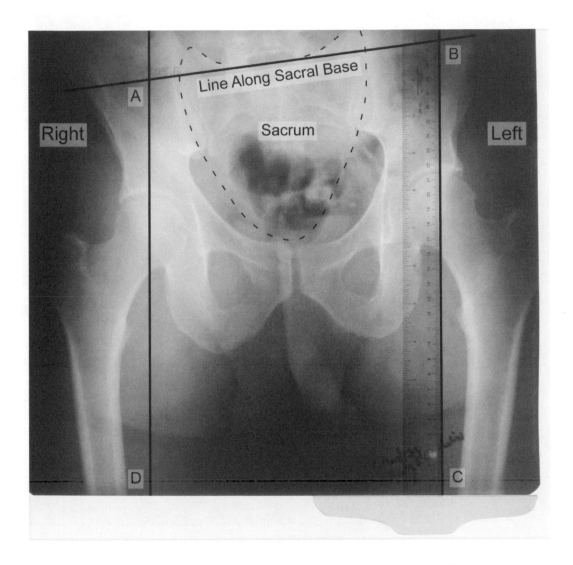

Fig. 16.1 — Using the "T" square to measure the length of line CB.

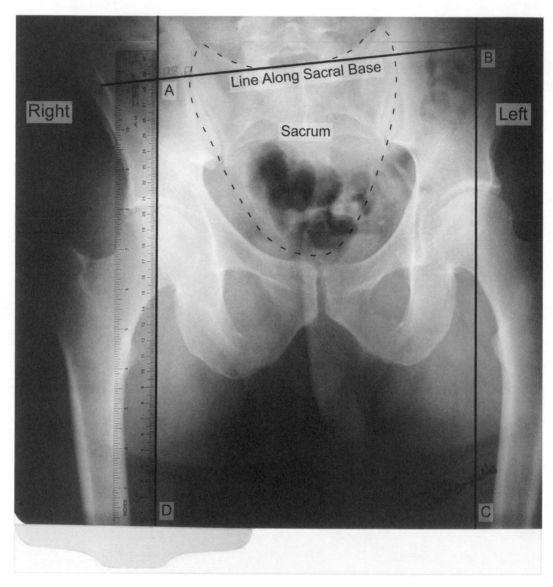

Fig. 16.2 — Same measurement is taken on the right side of the pelvis using line DA. Then simply compare the length of the two lines.

In Fig. 16.2, line CB measures 30.6 cm. Line DA, is 28.6 cm in length. That tells you that the left side of the pelvis is 30.6 cm -28.6 cm or 2.0 cm (20mm) higher than the right side. So, the patient would require a 2 cm lift for the right shoe *if* we wanted to *exactly* level the pelvis. (This example represents quite a large pelvic tilt.) I usually "pencil in" the length of each vertical line just above line AB (sacral base line) so that it is readily available for reference. It's that easy.

Now that the upright A-P is marked and measured, let's do the same with the upright LATERAL.

SEVENTEEN

Marking and Measuring the UPRIGHT LATERAL X-Ray

In addition to giving a good view of the sacral base, the lateral film can also give the health care professional other useful information, such as disc space height or thickness, the presence of vertebral degenerative changes, anterior-listhesis or retro-listhesis and the degree of lumbar lordosis. The degree of lumbar lordosis is given important consideration when deciding **how** to apply the lift correction. Let's now consider the lateral view from the perspective of pelvic tilt.

Using the UPRIGHT LATERAL view, we primarily want to assess the **sacral base angle** and the **degree of lumbar lordosis,** or how much backward curve the person has in the lumbar spine (Fig. 17.1). Determine this in the following manner:

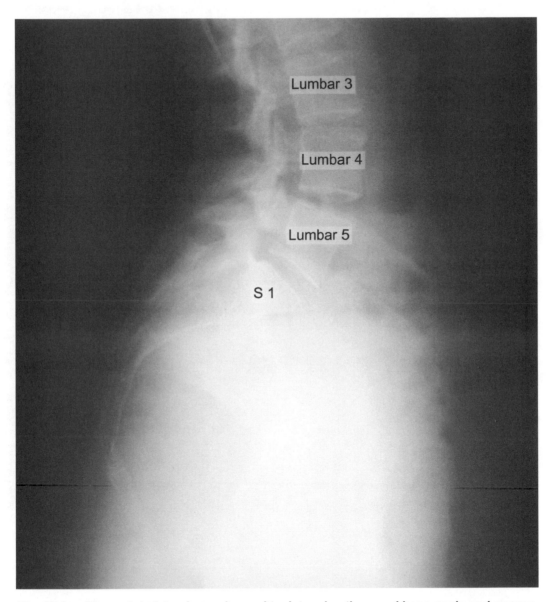

Fig. 17.1 — The upright lateral x-ray is used to determine the sacral base angle and assess the degree of lordosis (backward curve) present in the lumbar spine.

1. Draw a (pencil) line (AB) along the superior aspect (top) of the body of S1 and extend it for several inches in both directions. This line will slant, more or less, diagonally (Fig. 17.2 and Fig. 17.3).

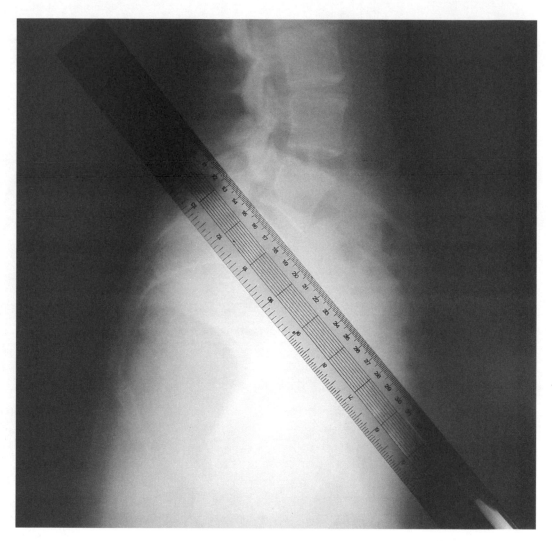

Fig. 17.2 — Place the straight edge along the top of the body of the 1st sacral vertebra (S1) and draw a line, AB, extending it for several inches in both directions.

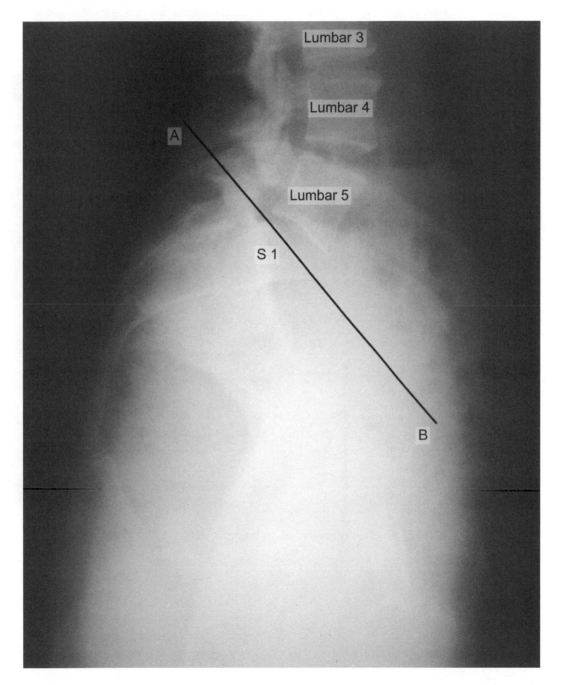

Fig. 17.3 — Shows line AB drawn along the top of the S1.

2. On this same line (AB), **at the most anterior aspect (front edge) of the body of S1,** make a small hash mark that crosses the line AB that you just drew (Fig. 17.4).

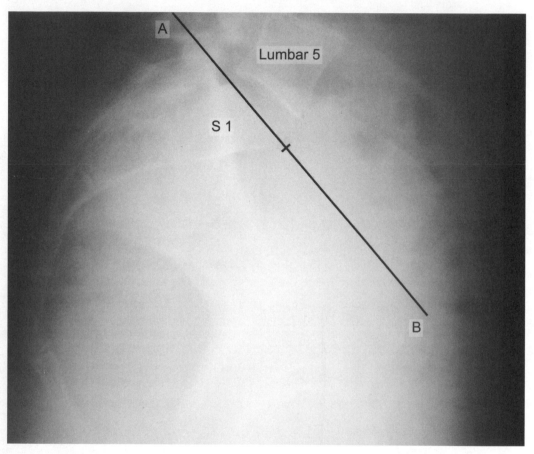

Fig. 17.4 — Shows a small hash mark that crosses line AB at the very front edge of the body of S1.

3. Draw a *horizontal* line (CD) that is *parallel to the bottom of the film.* This line should be several inches long and *pass through the junction made by line AB and the hash mark* (Fig. 17.5 and Fig. 17.6).

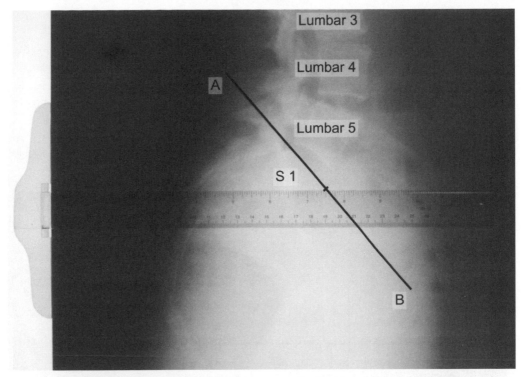

Fig. 17.5 — Using the "T" square to draw a line, CD, which is parallel to the bottom of the film and passes through the junction of line AB and the hash mark.

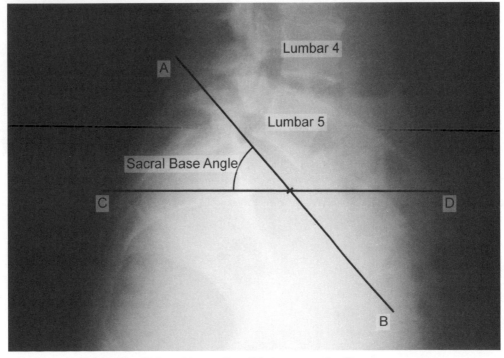

Fig. 17.6 — Shows line CD drawn on the film.
The intersection of lines AB and CD form the sacral base angle.

4. Using a protractor, measure the acute angle made by the above two lines (AB and CD). This is the **sacral base angle** (discussed below) (Fig. 17.7 and Fig. 17.8).

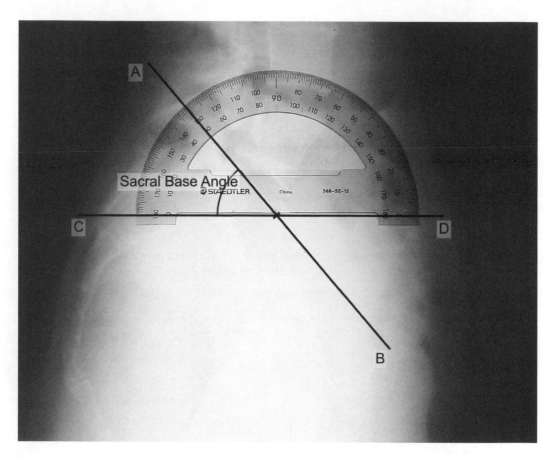

Fig. 17.7 — Using a protractor, measure the sacral base angle.

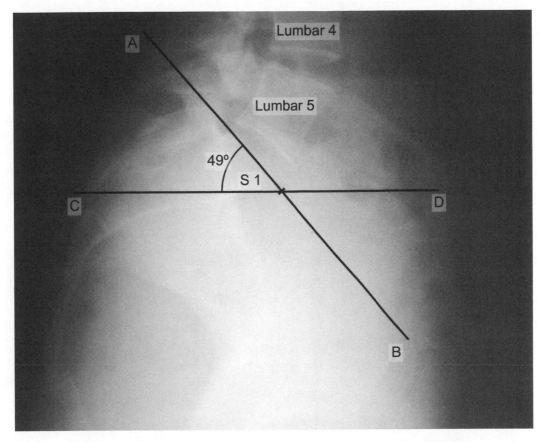

Fig. 17.8 — The sacral base angle measures 49 degrees in this person.

5. Place an easily visible dot in the middle of the body of L3 (Fig. 17.9) and drop a line (EF) *perpendicular* to the top edge of the film, down *through the dot* in the middle of the body of L3, toward the bottom of the film. Extend this line down below the line CD (Fig. 17.10 and Fig. 17.11). Line EF will usually pass through the body of the S1 vertebra in a person with a *normal* degree of lumbar lordosis.

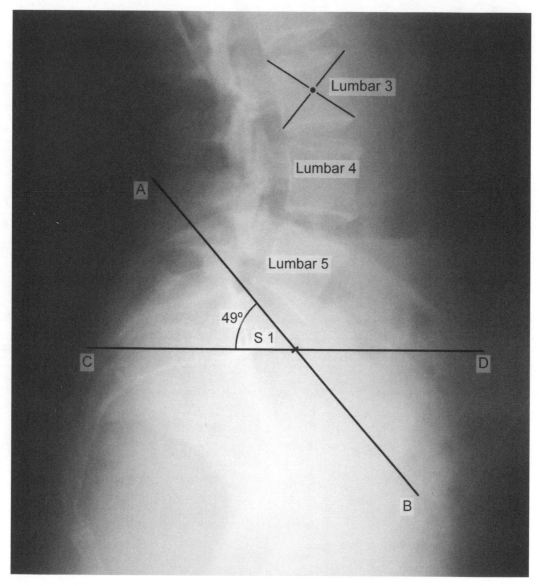

Fig. 17.9 — An easily visible dot is placed in the center of the body of the 3rd lumbar vertebra.

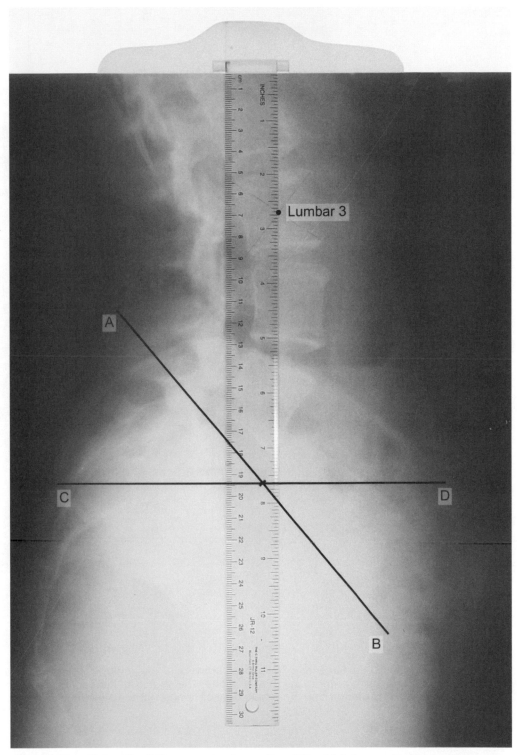

Fig. 17.10 — Using the "T" square to draw a line, EF, which is perpendicular to the top edge of the film, passes through the dot in the middle of the body of L3 and extends down below line CD.

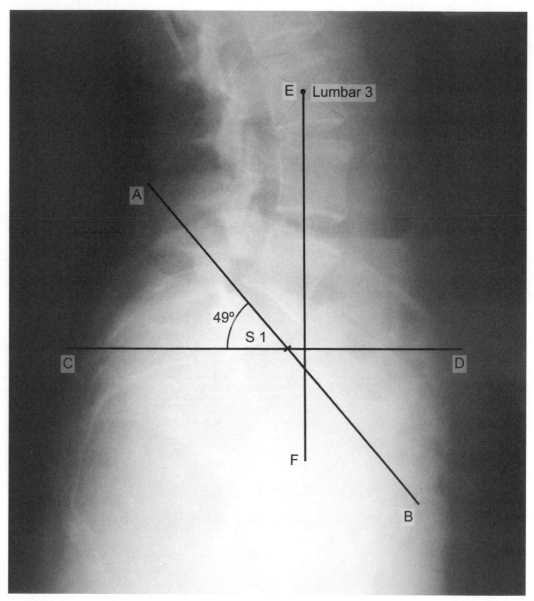

Fig. 17.11 — Shows all the necessary lines to be drawn and the angle to be measured on the upright lateral x-ray in order to accurately assess the degree of lumbar lordosis. This person has a greater than normal degree of lumbar lordosis (see text).

When viewed from the *side*, as in an UPRIGHT LATERAL x-ray of the pelvis, the entire sacrum can be seen to be *angled* or *tipped forward*. In other words, a side view of the sacrum shows that the *top* of the sacrum is *not level* with the horizon (Review Fig. 17.8). The degree to which the sacrum is tipped forward is measured as an angle called the sacral base angle. Generally speaking, the larger the **sacral base angle,** the greater the degree of lumbar lordosis, or backward curve, present in the lumbar spine.

In the LATERAL UPRIGHT x-ray of the pelvis, a normal sacral base angle is 40 (+/- 2 degrees). If the sacral base angle is greater than 42 degrees and if the perpendicular line from the body of L3 (line EF) passes anterior to (in front of) the body of S1, then there is a significant degree of lumbar lordosis present, as demonstrated in the x-ray of Fig. 17.11. The significance of a greater-than-normal degree of lordosis is this: It interferes with the free and easy motion of the lumbar spine and pelvis.

By prescribing a heel lift, we are, in effect, *increasing* the amount of lordotic curve in the lumbar spine by increasing the sacral base angle. If the UPRIGHT LATERAL x-ray of the patient *already* shows the presence of a significant amount of lordosis, we will want to keep this in mind and, perhaps, make modifications when applying the lift prescription. We will discuss **how** to do this later in more detail.

Congratulations! Now that you have successfully marked, measured, and analyzed an A-P AND LATERAL UPRIGHT film of the pelvis, it's time to prescribe the lift.

Summary

- Mark the upright lateral x-ray of the pelvis as in the chapter (Fig.17.11).

- The sacral base angle is a measure of to what degree the sacrum and, therefore, the entire pelvis, is tipped forward.

- A normal sacral base angle is 40 +/- 2 degrees.

- A larger than normal sacral base angle is often associated with an exaggeration of the normal backward curve in the lumbar spine (lumbar lordosis), which will cause line EF (Fig 17.11) to fall in front of the body of the first sacral vertebrae, S1.

- Any exaggeration of the normal lumbar lordosis becomes important in the application of the lift prescription.

EIGHTEEN

Prescribing the Lift

Prescribing a lift is easy if you follow a few simple guidelines. The actual amount of lift prescribed and how it is applied may vary from one health care professional to another due to differences in clinical experience and in preference. I will share what has worked for my patients and for me. The following are guidelines for the typical patient with a pelvic tilt and suggestions for the "not so typical" patient. They are meant to help if you come across a situation that is confusing to you. Don't get so caught up in the trees that you miss the forest. Most of the time, the simple, common sense approach will work.

ONE.

If you, the HCP, are skilled in manipulation techniques, it's a good idea to make sure that you restore as much free and easy motion as possible to the lumbar spine and pelvis *before* and *during* the application of the lift. Professionals not skilled in manipulation techniques should refer the patient to a favorite chiropractor, osteopath, physical therapist, naturopath or M.D. for appropriate manipulative care. Explain to the "manipulator" that the patient has a pelvic tilt and that you would like the patient examined, and, if necessary, treated for any dysfunction of the spine and pelvis. I would suggest weekly treatments continued at least until the patient has reached the final lift height, is pain-free and has good biomechanical motion of the lumbar spine and pelvis.

TWO.

Send the patient to physical therapy. Explain to the physical therapist that the patient has a pelvic tilt and request that (s)he work with **muscle-balancing techniques** and **stretching exercises** for the trunk, pelvis, and lower extremities, once weekly, before and during the process of applying the lift prescription. Continue at least until the final lift height is reached, the patient is pain-free and has good biomechanical motion of the spine and pelvis. Of course you—the HCP—may be perfectly capable of doing some or all of these things yourself. If so, GREAT! But, for the purpose of this discussion, I am assuming that you do *not* know how to do spinal manipulation or muscle-balancing techniques.

THREE.

In general, I like to prescribe the *least amount of lift correction* that will provide the patient with freedom from back pain *and* allow free and easy motion of the spine and pelvis upon examination. Simply put, I want to see good lumbar spine and pelvic bio-mechanics. Consider an example. If the A-P UPRIGHT x-ray shows a difference of 10mm (3/8-inch) between the two sides of the pelvis, I will start the patient out with a 1/4-inch lift in order to allow the pelvis time to adapt to a change in the tilt. I'll continue to treat the patient with manipulation and stretching or muscle- balancing exercises and observe. If the patient comes in for follow-up after having worn the lift for 4-6 weeks and reports (s)he's feeling well, I will examine the spine and pelvis to see if each is "moving" properly. If I see free and easy motion of the spine and pelvis, I may stop with the 1/4-inch lift. If the patient is *not* feeling better after several weeks of wearing the 1/4-inch lift *or* if my examination does not show free and easy motion of the spine and pelvis, I will increase the lift to the full 10mm (3/8-inch). If, of course, you are not doing the manipulation on the patient, rely on the "manipulator" to decide when good mechanics have been restored. Hence, the need for good communication among the health care team members.

FOUR.

Final Lift Prescription Between 5-9mm (3/16 to 3/8-inch)

If measurement of the UPRIGHT A-P x-ray of the pelvis calls **for a lift of anywhere between 5mm and 9mm (3/16- to 3/8-inch),** I will *usually* prescribe the entire lift prescription to be worn—at least temporarily—*inside* the heel portion of the shoe that corresponds to the lower side of the pelvis (refer to Figs. 11.1 and 11.2). In most cases, this will be satisfactory for the patient. In some instances, the lift may take up too much space inside of the shoe. In this situation, simply add the lift to the bottom of the heel on the outside of the shoe (Fig. 18.1). A skilled shoemaker can easily do this. When you and the patient are satisfied with the final lift prescription, it's the patient's decision, based on comfort and convenience, as to whether the lift is worn inside or on the bottom of the shoe.

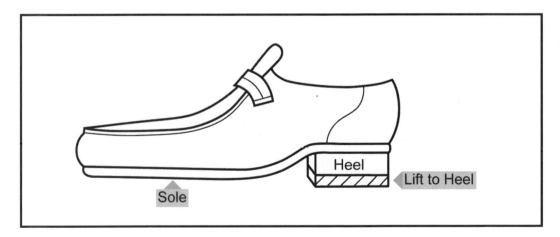

Fig. 18.1 — Shows how a lift may be added to the bottom of the heel of a shoe. Any shoemaker can easily do this.

FIVE.

Most people can tolerate the addition of up to a 3/8-inch lift with no problem. For elderly people or those who are very sedentary or very stiff with regard to the musculo-skeletal system, one may certainly *begin* with 1/4-inch and increase it later to 3/8-inch as discussed above. However, if the patient has a *very large* degree of lumbar lordosis (as indicated by a sacral base angle of around 50 degrees or greater and the perpendicular line (EF) from the center of the body of L3 passing anterior to the body of S1), (Fig. 17.11), then you might want to "divide" the 3/8-inch lift between the heel and sole of the appropriate shoe (discussed below).

SIX.

Final Lift Prescription Greater Than 3/8-inch Up To 1/2-inch (10-13mm)

With regard to **a lift that is greater than 3/8-inch and up to 1/2-inch,** one finds that many patients do not like to wear a lift of that size (1/2-inch) inside the shoe, because it takes up too much room. With a lift of this size, consider applying the lift in an alternative manner. If the final lift prescription is *closer to 1/2-inch,* add the lift to the bottom of the heel of the appropriate shoe in the patient with a *normal* degree of lumbar lordosis, or "divide" the lift between the heel and the sole of the shoe of the patient with an *exaggerated* degree of lumbar lordosis.

By "dividing" the lift between the heel and the sole of the shoe, the patient has some options that can make wearing the lift safer and more comfortable.

Remember that a heel lift of any size *increases* the lumbar lordosis to some degree. So, if your patient has:

- a sacral base angle of greater than 42 degrees, *and*

- the perpendicular line dropped from the middle of the body of L3 falls anterior to the body of S1, *and*

- the patient requires a lift prescription of *close to 1/2-inch,* then, you can "divide" the lift. The division can be done in either of the following ways:

1. For a total lift of 1/2-inch, add *half* of the lift prescription (in this case 1/4-inch) to the *entire sole* of the appropriate shoe, then add the *other half* of the lift prescription (1/4-inch) to *just the heel* of the same shoe (Fig. 18.2). This way, the heel will be lifted 1/2-inch, yet, the difference between the heel of the shoe and the sole of the shoe is only 1/4-inch. Thus, the lordosis will only be increased minimally. This alteration also interferes less with the mechanics of walking. Think about it and you'll understand.

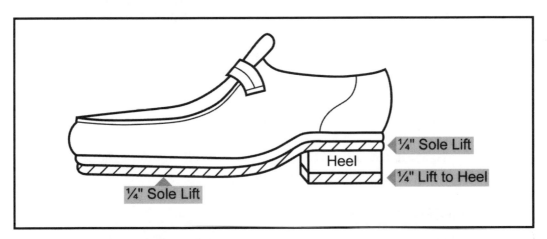

Fig. 18.2 — Demonstrates one method of "dividing" the lift prescription: placing half of the thickness of the lift prescription on the entire sole of the shoe and the other half on just the heel portion of the shoe.

2. Another option, which essentially does the same thing, is to add *half* of the lift prescription as a *partial sole* to the bottom of the shoe that corresponds to the *lower* side of the pelvis. Then add the *full* lift prescription to *just the heel* portion of the same shoe. For example, if the lift prescription is for a

total of 1/2-inch, add 1/4-inch as a partial sole and add 1/2-inch to the heel of the same shoe (Fig. 18.3).

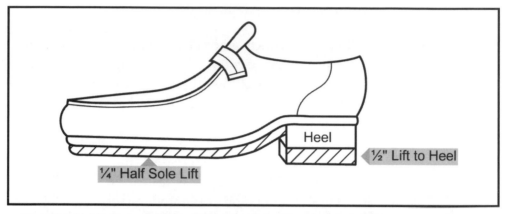

Fig. 18.3 — Another method of "dividing" the lift prescription: Place half of the thickness of the lift prescription as a partial sole on the shoe and place the full thickness of the lift prescription on just the heel portion of the shoe.

"Dividing" the lift is easier, of course, if the patient wears shoes that already come with a heel, like dress shoes or boots. For other types of shoes, see below.

SEVEN.

As we discussed earlier, emphasize that the patient should wear the lift *all the time*, at home or away.

EIGHT.

The body may take from three to 16 weeks to adjust to the addition of a lift, even one as small as 1/4-inch. Be patient. The patient may complain of the same lower back symptoms for several weeks. If the patient faithfully wears the lift, does manipulation, muscle balancing, and stretching exercises, the odds are that one day soon, the patient will walk in and say that (s)he is feeling better.

NINE.

Final Lift Prescription Greater Than 1/2-inch

If the x-ray calls **for a total lift of greater than 1/2-inch up to 3/4-inch or even higher**—the basic principles already discussed apply. Divide the lift between the heel and sole of the shoe as outlined (review Figs. 18.2 & 18.3).

TEN.

A skilled shoemaker can seamlessly incorporate a lift into the sole and/or heel of practically any type of shoe, even a "sneaker" type shoe or Birkenstocks (Fig. 18.4 and Fig. 18.5). Many people will ask you about this because these shoes are so popular. Make the acquaintance of your friendly, neighborhood shoemaker. I appreciate mine very much.

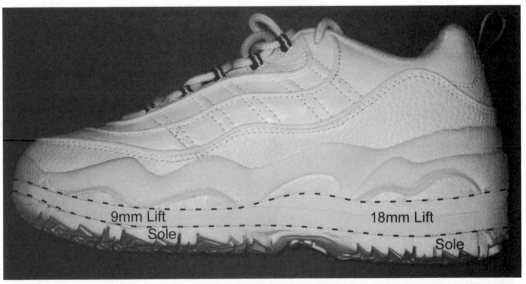

Fig. 18.4 — Shows how a sneaker-type shoe can be modified to accommodate a lift. Notice that the sole has been removed and the lift inserted. Then the sole was, again, glued onto the bottom of the shoe. This example shows an 18mm lift in the heel portion of the shoe, tapering down to a 9mm lift on the sole.

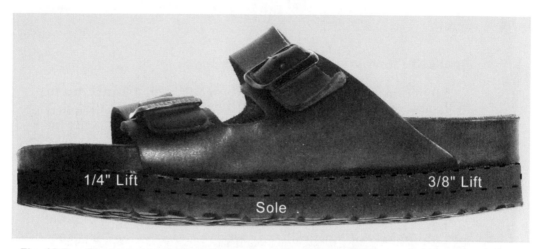

Fig. 18.5 — Shows how a Birkenstock-type shoe may be modified. Again, the sole was removed, the lift inserted and the sole reapplied. Here there is a 3/8-inch lift in the heel tapering down to 1/4-inch in the sole.

These guidelines and suggestions should be useful to you. You will more fully understand them after you have treated a few patients. For now, please accept them on good faith. Refer to them frequently and don't be afraid to put these concepts into use. Jump in, follow the guidelines and do it. You'll find it is easy and follows common sense. You'll be comfortable with a lift prescription in no time at all.

Summary

1. For a final lift prescription up to 3/8-inch (9-10mm), use a lift inside the heel portion of the shoe or add it to the bottom of the heel of the shoe, as dictated by patient comfort/preference. For patients with a very large degree of lumbar lordosis, divide the lift as follows: add 3/8-inch to the heel portion of the shoe, tapering the lift down to 1/4-inch along the sole (review Fig. 18.2 through Fig. 18.5).

2. For a final lift prescription from 3/8-inch to 1/2-inch (9/10 to 12/13mm), consider adding the lift to the bottom of the heel for better shoe fit, or divide the lift between the heel and the sole on the bottom of the shoe as outlined above, especially if the patient has an exaggerated lumbar lordosis.

3. For a final lift prescription greater than 1/2-inch (12/13mm), divide the lift between the heel and sole on the bottom of the shoe.

NINETEEN

Monitoring the Patient

How can we monitor the patient's progress during the phases of lift prescription, manipulation, muscle balancing and stretching exercises?

GENERAL

If the HCP is not skilled in manipulation and muscle-balancing techniques, treating the patient with a pelvic tilt is a collaborative effort. All members of the team should get to know each other: chiropractor, physical therapist, osteopath, M.D., naturopath, massage therapist, sports trainer or exercise physiologist. The goal should be to help the patient. Good communication is the key. Leave egos at the door.

1. If the primary HCP is the person doing the manipulation, I suggest that you see the patient once weekly for evaluation and treatment. Remember, it takes time for the pelvis to adapt to the application of a lift. Manipulation and stretching exercises are very helpful during this adaptation phase. If the primary HCP is not the person doing the manipulation, I suggest seeing the patient every two-three weeks. However, the patient should have manipulation and, if needed, muscle-balancing once per week. The stretching exercises should be done daily (see Chapter Twenty-Three).

2. On the first visit after having prescribed the lift, *visually inspect and measure* the lift to see that the patient is wearing the exact thickness prescribed and is wearing it in the correct shoe. Make sure it's made of either firm, non-compressible rubber or hard leather (preferred) like the kind of leather that one finds as soles on the bottoms of shoes.

3. Determine if the lift is *comfortable*. Sometimes, a hard leather lift causes heel pain. If this is the case, either change to a hard rubber lift, which is softer, or simply put the lift on the bottom of the shoe instead of inside the shoe. If the patient wears sneaker/athletic shoes and wants to wear the lift inside the shoe, the lift can often be placed under the insole of the shoe for added comfort. Lifts up to 1/4-inch can even be worn *inside* the heel portion of Birkenstocks. The patient should change the lift (get a new one) every 8-12 months.

4. Ask the patient how (s)he is feeling since the last visit. Inquire as to the exact location of any pain. If someone else is doing the manipulation, ask about how that has been going for the patient. If the patient is seeing a physical therapist for muscle-balancing, inquire about that, too. Specifically ask if there has been any noticeable improvement or worsening in any daily activities like walking, sitting, standing, and sleeping.

5. Have the patient perform the exercises that were prescribed by you or the therapist and note:

   A. whether they are being done correctly, and

   B. the ease/difficulty that the patient has when the patient is doing them.

   From week to week, you can actually see the patient's progress.

6. Review the A-P UPRIGHT and LATERAL x-rays as a reminder of the degree of pelvic tilt and the degree of lumbar lordosis. Reviewing all of the above information and the x-rays helps the HCP decide whether changes need to be made in the lift prescription or to leave it alone.

7. When the patient says that (s)he is feeling significantly better and the "manipulator" and the "muscle balancer" agree that there has been significant improvement in spinal and pelvic mechanics, then you have done your job well. You will have a very grateful patient.

   But what happens if the patient is not showing any improvement after 10-16 weeks?

TWENTY

Troubleshooting

If the patient is not showing at least some improvement 10-16 weeks after the *final* lift prescription has been applied, ask the following questions:

A. Have the patient's x-rays been accurately marked and accurately measured?

B. Has the lift prescription been properly applied, taking into account all of the suggestions discussed, especially with regard to increased lumbar lordosis?

C. Has the patient been wearing the lift *all the time*?

D. Has the patient been doing the stretching/muscle balancing exercises *correctly* and *regularly*?

If the answer to *any* of these questions is "no," correct what needs to be corrected. *Any one* of the above, *by itself,* can prevent the patient from improving.

If the answer to *all* of these questions is "yes," then it's time to:

1. Request a new UPRIGHT A-P x-ray of the pelvis. This time, have the x-ray taken with the patient's *shoes on and the lift in place.*

2. Compare this x-ray with the initial UPRIGHT A-P taken with the patient barefoot. See if there has been enough correction provided by the lift already prescribed. This second x-ray, taken with shoes and lift in place, should demonstrate the pelvis to be within 4-5mm of being level. Sometimes, especially in big people, the body weight is enough to compress the lift so much that it does not provide enough correction. If this is the case, you will be able to see it on the repeat x-ray and you may have to add more lift. Recheck after 4-6 weeks. The patient should continue with the manipulation, the stretching exercises, and the physical therapy during this time.

3. Consult with the person doing the manipulation and with the person doing the muscle balancing. If one or both say that there is still work to be done, then you have an answer to the question as to why the patient isn't better yet. But, if the "manipulator" tells you that normal lumbar and pelvic mechanics have been restored, the physical therapist says that the patient has good muscle balance and is flexible and the UPRIGHT A-P x-ray shows adequate lift correction (to within 4-5mm of level), then there are more things to consider (see #4 below).

4. Make certain that other causes of a failed lower back syndrome have not been overlooked, namely:

   A. Dysfunction of the lower thoracic and lumbar spine, especially when the vertebra is in a flexed position.

   B. Pubic symphysis dysfunction

   C. Posterior nutation or posterior torsion of the sacrum

   D. Shear dysfunction of the innominate (hip) bone

5. Double check to make sure that the patient does not have other, more serious medical (or surgical) causes of lower back pain (tumor, fracture, infection, herniated disk, and spinal stenosis).

6. Have the patient continue to wear the lift and continue to do the stretching exercises daily. Some patients respond more slowly and may require *up to six months or more* of wearing the final lift prescription and stretching before they start to feel better. This is often true of patients who have a large lift prescription (greater than 1/2-inch), and especially in people who lack flexibility in the lumbar spine and lower extremities. Have the patient continue with the manipulation, once every week or two, during the following six months. *Some people just take longer than expected to get better.* Over and over, experience has shown me that most people will get better with correct application of these tried and true principles, persistent and regular effort in doing the stretching exercises, and a healthy dose of "tincture of time."

7. Unfortunately, sometimes patients just don't get better, in spite of the HCP's best efforts. With proper lift prescription, manipulation, stretching and muscle-balancing exercises, one can expect that approximately 70% of persons with a failed lower back syndrome that includes a pelvic tilt will get better. That's pretty good, though, considering that most of these people were told they were going to have to live with their pain for the rest of their lives.

8. It is strongly recommended that the patient continue to wear the lift, even if (s)he has not obtained the relief that was hoped for. A level pelvis has a very beneficial effect on the hip joints, knee joints and joints of the lumbar spine and pelvis by reducing the stress on them and thereby reducing the wear and tear that occurs over time.

TWENTY-ONE

Side Effects of Lift Therapy

The most common side effect of lift therapy is pain of some kind. This most commonly occurs in the heel and foot, but occasionally in the ankle and knee, and even in the hip and lower back. If the pain is in the heel, the foot, ankle, or the knee, assume it is due to a change in the mechanics of walking caused by the lift. An aggravation of hip and lower back pain is almost always caused by the *change in the tilt of the pelvis* due to the lift. This occasionally happens in the early stages of wearing a lift as the pelvis begins to adapt to the change brought about by the lift. This is not necessarily a bad sign.

Most of the time, the aggravation of hip and lower back pain will disappear within two to three weeks after the lift has been applied, especially if the person is doing manipulation, stretching exercises, and muscle-balancing. If the hip and lower back pain persist, reduce the size of the lift temporarily, or ask the person to wear the lift intermittently for a while. For example, if the person is wearing a 3/8-inch lift, drop it to 1/4-inch and ask them to wear the lift for just a few hours per day. Soon thereafter, increase the time it is worn, as tolerated, until (s)he is able to wear the 1/4-inch lift all the time. Increase the lift back up to 3/8-inch, if indicated. These remedies are usually successful in eliminating the aggravation of hip and lower back pain.

Heel pain is by far the most common of the side effects. This occurs most often in patients who choose to wear the lift inside the shoe rather than outside on the bottom of the heel of the shoe. The first thing to do to correct this is to change the lift from hard leather to **hard** rubber, which is slightly softer. This will often solve the problem. If this doesn't help, suggest that the patient have the lift put on the bottom of the heel of the shoe. This almost always eliminates heel pain. If the patient wears the lift inside an athletic/sneaker shoe, putting it under the insole of the sneaker will often make it much more comfortable.

If complaints of heel pain continue, even if the patient is wearing the lift on the bottom of the shoe and the principles of lift application have been properly followed, then consider the use of an orthotic inside the shoe. In other words, an orthotic can take the pressure off the heel and distribute it more evenly throughout the foot. Perhaps at this time, a podiatry consult would be in order. *Remember to take the thickness of the orthotic into consideration. It will count as part or all of the lift prescription.* To go this route, good communication between the HCP and the podiatrist is essential.

Request that the podiatrist do one of two things:

A. If the lift prescription is small enough (1/4-inch), it *may be possible* to incorporate the lift into the orthotic.

or

B. If the lift prescription is greater than 1/4-inch, the patient can wear the orthotic inside the shoe and add the lift separately to the bottom of the shoe according to the principles outlined in Chapter Eighteen.

After the patient is fitted with the orthotic, a new UPRIGHT A-P x-ray should be taken with the shoes on and the orthortic and lift in place. Compare this new x-ray with the original barefooted x-rays and make any changes in the lift prescription that might be indicated because of the orthotic. Don't assume that the orthotic has been made as requested.

Another less common side effect is ipsilateral ankle or knee pain. Adding the lift to the bottom of the shoe—and especially by dividing the lift between the heel and the sole—will usually prevent or correct this. Also, ask the HCP doing manipulation to look at the knee or ankle. Simple manipulation of the joint may be all that is needed.

One potential problem should be addressed. Whenever a lift is added to the bottom of a shoe, whether it is added to just the heel or to both the heel and the sole, be sure to advise the patient to be extra careful. It is surprising how *unconsciously* we live. We automatically take into account the thickness of our shoes while going about our daily activities, such as walking, going up or down stairs, stepping over things, etc. With the addition of a lift to just one shoe, it's easy to miscalculate, misstep, trip, and fall when you have an extra 1/4-inch to 3/4-inch "sticking out" from the bottom of one shoe. For obvious reasons, this can be of great importance to our senior patients. A reminder to the patient to be extra careful is very appropriate.

TWENTY-TWO

Introduction to Stretching Exercises

If I were to spend the next ten hours emphasizing the importance of stretching and flexibility as they relate to lower back pain, it would be time well spent. Many of my patients with a history of chronic low back pain do *not* have a pelvic tilt and, therefore, do *not* need to wear a lift. These patients will often get better with manipulation and stretching exercises. My patients who regularly do the exercises that I prescribe are often very pleased with their progress.

Often ignored, stretching exercises are a very *important* part of getting better. My experience is that, in general, most people are as stiff as a board. This is true not only for those who lead a sedentary life, but also for those who are athletically inclined. I know several people who have great cardiovascular endurance and tremendous physical strength and cannot touch their toes. I am amazed that they are surprised that they have back pain. When it comes to having a pain-free musculo-skeletal system, flexibility is a key factor.

One of the main jobs of muscles is to move joints. If the muscles, tendons and ligaments that are connected to specific joints are tight— like the lumbar spine joints or sacro-iliac joints—then you will experience stiffness and restricted or limited motion when you try to move those joints. If you try to move *beyond* the stretching capacity of those tight muscles, tendons and ligaments that connect to those joints, you will feel pain, and possibly even muscle spasm. Tight muscles are a *very common* cause of back pain. The muscles gradually get tighter with age, sedentary lifestyle and lack of stretching.

A typical story is this. A person is out working in the yard in the spring after a long winter of relative inactivity. (S)he bends over to pick up a basket of weeds and WHAM!!! The lower back muscles are stretched beyond their usual capacity. The muscles immediately go into spasm and the person is unable to move. If, on the other hand, you stay flexible by stretching daily, you will avoid many musculo-skeletal problems in the future.

I *always* give my patients stretching exercises to do at home. Although I always tailor the exercises to suit the individual situation, there are some of the basic ones I like. Again, I would like to emphasize their importance. *The stretching exercises are just as important as the lift, the manipulation, and the muscle balancing.*

> ## CAUTION!
>
> ### DO NOT ATTEMPT TO DO ANY OF THESE EXERCISES WITHOUT FIRST GETTING THE OKAY FROM YOUR HEALTH CARE PROFESSIONAL!!

GENERAL

1. Take these exercises seriously. Respect them as you would any medication that you have been prescribed. Do not underestimate their ability to help you if you do them properly and carefully.

2. Exercise regularly. Set aside a period of time every day to exercise. If you are very stiff in the morning, even after a hot bath or shower, you may wait until later in the day before beginning to do these exercises, when your body has had a chance to loosen up a little. *Gradually*, work up to the point where you are able to do as many of the exercises as you can, twice daily.

3. Wear loose-fitting clothes that will accommodate stretching.

4. Do the exercises slowly and carefully and with attention. *Feel* what is happening in your body and *where* it is happening while you are doing each exercise. Don't try to cram them into your already rushed morning schedule. Get up earlier so that you can give them the time and the attention they (and you) require.

5. *If you have a problem with a particular exercise, stop doing the exercise until you tell your HCP about it.* You may have difficulty distinguishing between the discomfort of stretching something that hasn't been stretched in a long time (soft tissue) and joint pain. However, it's usually just soft tissue that hasn't been stretched in a long time.

6. You may feel stiff and sore for a few days after you begin the exercise program, especially if you are not used to physical activity. Don't be discouraged. Most likely, you're doing a little too much, too soon. You may want to shorten the length of time that you do each exercise or take a couple of days off until you feel better. Check it out with your HCP. If you get the okay to resume, do so.

7. *Be patient with yourself. Stretching out body parts that haven't been stretched for years takes time.*

8. I have offered an alternative to many of the exercises. Those who cannot do a particular exercise can try the alternative(s).

9. If you *are able* to do the primary exercise, you *do not have* to do the alternative exercises (although you are encouraged to do all of them if you can). The alternative exercises are for those of you who, *for any reason,* are not able to do the main exercise.

10. *Do not do any of the exercises that are too difficult for you to perform.* Most people can do at least some of these exercises. If these exercises are too difficult to do, ask your HCP to refer you to a physical therapist. The therapist will help you with these exercises or prescribe ones that you *can* do that will have a similar effect. Don't try to be "macho" and hurt yourself. The goal is to feel *better*, not macho.

11. Refer to the photographs frequently, especially when first trying the exercises, to be sure you are doing them correctly.

12. Doing stretching exercises is a form of physical therapy. Stretching muscles, tendons and ligaments that are not used to being stretched can be *work*, plain and simple. Once you decide which ones are better for you, set up a daily regimen and be disciplined. Keep your goal in mind: a flexible, pain-free lower back. This will help to keep you on task.

13. Read through *all* the exercises and look at *all* of the photos *before* attempting to *do* them. This will give you an idea of which ones you think you can do and which ones may be too difficult.

14. Read the above items *again*, especially the **"CAUTION"** at the top.

TWENTY-THREE

Specific Exercises

EXERCISE 1

STARTING POSITION

Sit on the floor with your legs loosely crossed in front of you. Drop your chin to your chest and keep it there. Place your hands on the

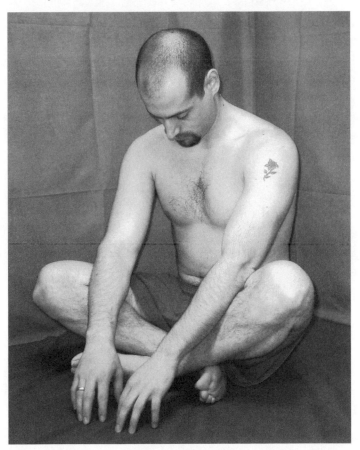

Fig. 23.1 — Exercise 1, starting position. Key points are: chin on chest, breathe easy, muscles relaxed.

floor in front of your legs (Fig. 23.1). Breathe freely and easily. Don't hold your breath.

ACTION

Notice whether you feel tightness in your body and, if so, where? Bend forward, *using your lower back vertebrae to bend,* until you feel a good stretch. Don't keep your lower back straight. Bend it forward! You may feel the stretch anywhere from your neck down to your hips, and even to your knees. Where you feel the stretch is where you have a restriction. Relax into this restriction until it "releases." Stop at this point and ask yourself the following questions:

- Is my chin on my chest?

- Am I relaxed?

- Am I breathing freely and easily?

If not, make it so. *Do not bend forward any farther until you have relaxed into your present position.* Feel the stretch, stay relaxed, and allow the breath to come in and go out as it wants to. *Only* when you feel reasonably comfortable in that position, bend forward a little bit more until you again feel a good stretch. Then stop and ask yourself the same questions as above. Your goal, in time, is to be able to place your elbows and forearms on the floor in front of you with your chin on your chest, your muscles relaxed, and your breathing free and easy (Fig. 23.2). The entire exercise should take three minutes. During this time, you should go as far as you can *comfortably* go and then stay in that position until the three minutes have passed.

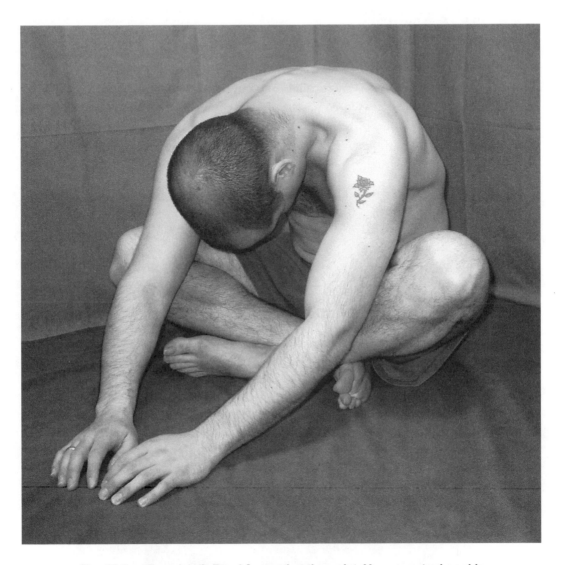

Fig. 23.2 — Exercise 1. Bend forward at the waist. Your eventual goal is to be able to stretch forward enough to place your elbows, forearms and hands on the floor in front of you.

ALTERNATIVE TO EXERCISE 1

STARTING POSITION

This alternative exercise is for those of you who have pain in the knees when trying to bend your knees in the above exercise. It is also for those whose "stomach" gets in the way and prevents you from bending forward when your legs are crossed. Instead of crossing your legs, place your legs in front of you at approximately a 30-degree angle with knees slightly bent (Fig. 23.3). Place your chin on your chest. Breathe freely and easily. Relax.

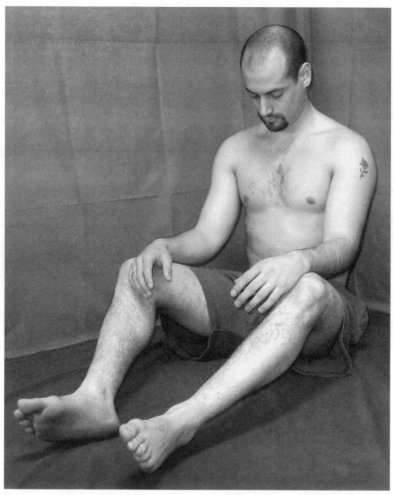

Fig. 23.3 — Alternative to Exercise 1, starting position. Key points are: chin on chest; breathe easy and relax your muscles.

ACTION

Bend forward at the waist, using your lower lumbar vertebrae. If you are able, grasp your big toes with your index fingers and thumbs, so that you have something to hold on to (Fig. 23.4). If you have to bend your knees a little more toward you in order to grab your toes, that's okay. Keep your arms and hands between your knees. Drop your chin to your chest. Hold on and feel the stretch in your lower back. Stay in this position and breathe easy for 30-60 seconds, allowing yourself to adapt to this posture.

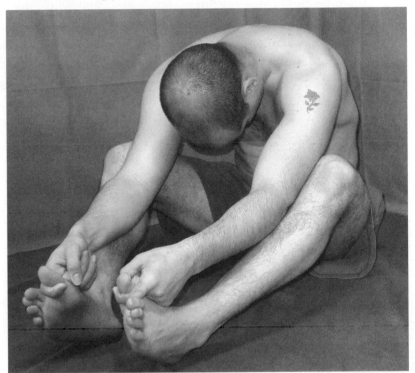

Fig. 23.4 — Alternative to Exercise 1. Grabbing your toes gives you something to hold on to. Gradually straightening out your legs, as tolerated, will increase the stretch.

When you feel as if you have relaxed into this position, straighten out your legs (knees) a little bit more, still holding on to your toes, until you again feel a good stretch. You may feel the stretch anywhere from your neck to your ankles. Continue in this manner until two or three minutes have elapsed. The goal is to hold on to your toes and straighten out your legs as much as you *comfortably* can in the allotted time. If you can eventually get your elbows to touch your knees with your legs (knees) straight, you're doing *very* well. This stretch will be useful for those who are unable to sit in a cross-legged position.

EXERCISE 2

STARTING POSITION

Sit on the floor with your legs extended (out in front of you). Place your chin on your chest. Straighten your legs so that your knees are *gently* locked. If you cannot straighten out your knees completely, then place a pillow or a towel under them. Point your feet and toes toward the ceiling. Elbows and forearms should be placed on your thighs and *remain in contact with the thighs* throughout the entire exercise (Fig. 23.5). Breathe easy.

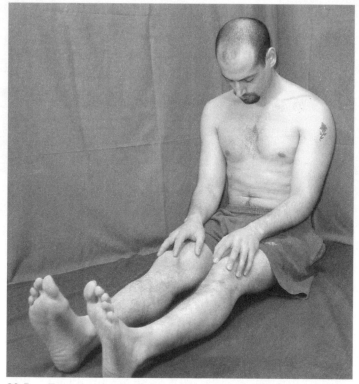

Fig. 23.5 — Exercise 2, starting position. Key points are: chin on chest; knees straight; feet pointing toward the ceiling; elbows, forearms and hands in contact with the thighs. Relax and breathe easy.

ACTION

You may *already* feel a good stretch, anywhere from your neck to your calves. If so, stay relaxed, breathe freely and easily and notice where you feel the stretch. Stay in this position until you feel comfortable. Then bend forward at the waist, sliding your forearms forward along your thighs until you feel a good stretch. As you bend forward, remember to keep your chin on your chest (Fig. 23.6). When you feel the tightness, notice where it is. This is where you are restricted. Stay in this position, breathe freely and easily with your chin on your chest until you feel as if you have relaxed into this new position. Continue like this until three minutes have passed. Your *eventual* goal is to be able to bend forward enough so that your elbows can reach your knees.

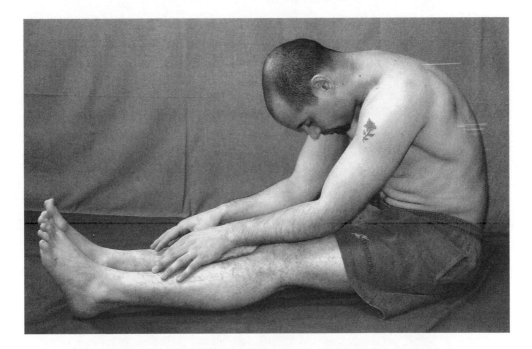

Fig. 23.6 — Exercise 2. Slide your elbows, forearms and hands down along your thighs and legs as you bend forward at the waist.

ALTERNATIVE #1 TO EXERCISE 2

STARTING POSITION

Many people, because of stiffness, are unable to even sit in the starting position of exercise 2. In other words, they are not even able to sit on the floor with their trunk and legs at a 90-degree angle. If this is true for you, I suggest the following alternative exercise. You will need a sash, a belt, towel or a rope for this exercise. Sit on a pillow or a towel (optional) on the floor, so that your pelvis is tilted slightly forward. Place your legs out in front of you. Hold one end of the belt in each hand. Place the middle or center portion of the belt around the balls of your feet. You may wish to wrap a portion of the belt or sash around your hands to give you a better grip. You may also start with your knees slightly bent, and then straighten them out as you loosen up (Fig. 23.7). Drop your chin to your chest.

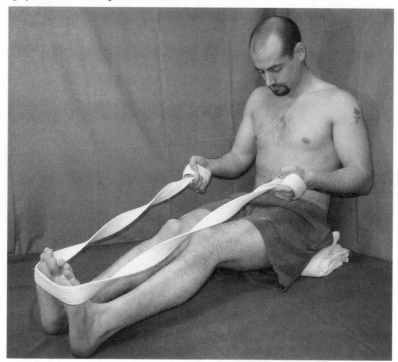

Fig. 23.7 — Alternative 1 to Exercise 2, starting position. For persons who are unable to sit up straight with legs out in front of them, the use of a sash, belt, towel or a rope will be very helpful.

ACTION

Bending your lower back, pull yourself *gently* forward, until you feel a good stretch in your lower back and in the backs of your thighs, knees, and calves. When you feel a good stretch, stop at that point and relax into it. Take up any slack in the sash or belt by wrapping it around your hands, so that your arms are straight or slightly bent at the elbows. Breathe freely and easily. After you have relaxed into that position, bend forward and pull yourself a little bit farther forward until you again feel a good stretch. This is a two to three minute exercise. Your goal, in time, is to be able to pull yourself forward at the waist and slide your forearms down along your thighs until your elbows can reach your knees with your knees straight (Fig. 23.8).

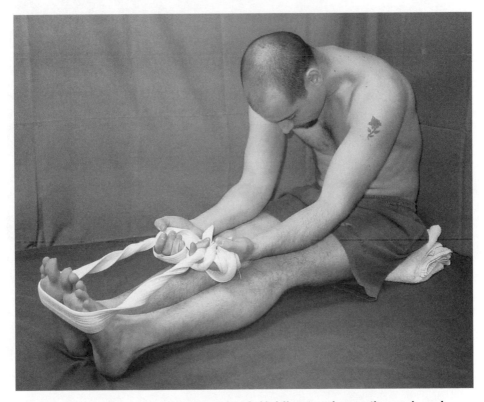

Fig. 23.8 — Alternative 1 to Exercise 2. Holding tension on the sash and with knees as straight as possible, gradually pull yourself forward at the waist until you feel a good stretch.
Try to keep elbows and forearms in contact with your thighs.

ALTERNATIVE #2 TO EXERCISE 2

STARTING POSITION

This exercise is for persons who have too much back pain or too big of a "stomach" when trying to bend forward at the waist to do the previous exercise. This exercise allows you to rest your back and, at the same time, stretch your hamstring muscles and calves. Use a belt, a sash, a rope, or a towel with this exercise. Sit on the floor with both legs out in front of you. Place the belt around the ball of one of your feet (Fig. 23.9). Then, lie flat on your back on the floor and pull

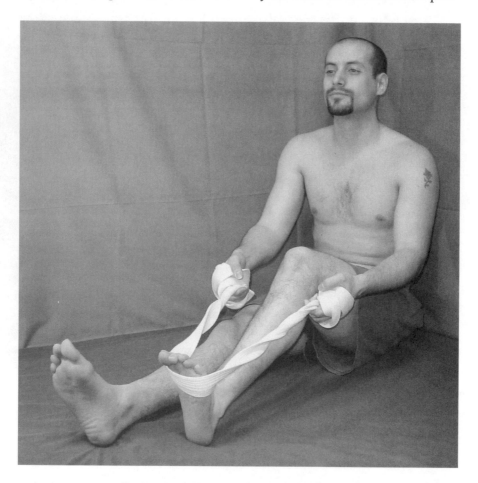

Fig. 23.9 — Alternative 2 to Exercise 2, starting position. While keeping one leg straight, slightly bend the other knee and place the sash around the ball of the foot. Keep slight tension on the sash.

the thigh to a 90-degree angle with your trunk. Leave the other leg lying flat on the floor (Fig. 23.10). You may use a pillow for your head or opposite knee, if desired.

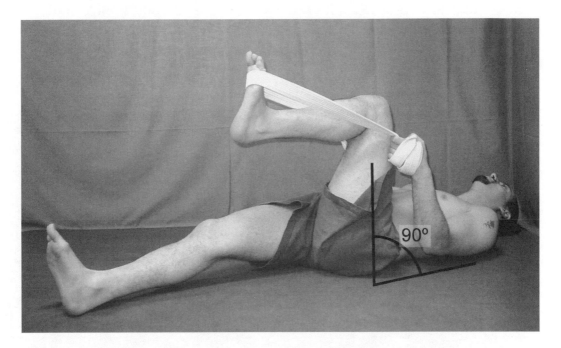

Fig. 23.10 — Alternative 2 to Exercise 2. Key points: lie flat on your back with your head on the floor and relax; keep tension on the sash; make certain that your trunk and your thigh are at 90 degrees to each other.

ACTION

With your thigh at 90-degrees to your trunk and keeping tension on the rope/belt, slowly straighten out the knee joint until you feel a gentle stretch in your hamstring muscle (Fig. 23.11). Hold this stretch for 10-15 seconds. Then bend the knee slightly to release the stretch. Repeat this stretch several times until you can hold the stretch for about 30 seconds at a time. Your *eventual* goal is to be able to straighten out the knee with the thigh at 90-degrees to your trunk. Remember to stretch the other leg, too.

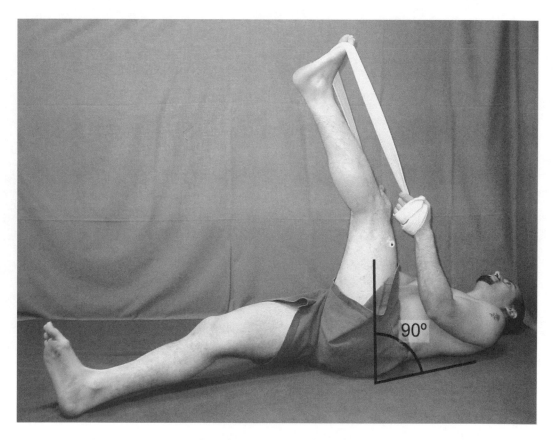

Fig. 23.11 — Alternative 2 to Exercise 2. Keeping tension on the sash, slowly straighten out your leg until you feel a good stretch in your hamstring muscle. You may also feel a stretch in your calf. Keep your head on the floor and keep your trunk and thigh at 90 degrees.

EXERCISE 3

STARTING POSITION

Sit on a stool, chair, or bench with a 90-degree angle between your trunk and your thighs and a 90-degree angle between your thighs and your legs. Place either ankle on top of the opposite knee. Put your chin on your chest. Place both hands on the shin bone (Fig. 23.12). If the chair is too high for you, place some books under your foot, so that your ankle doesn't slide off your knee.

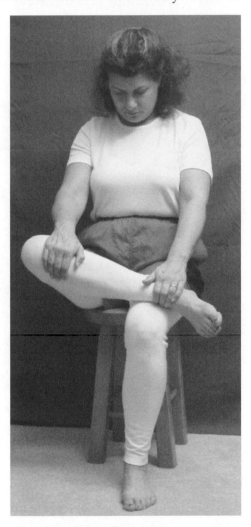

Fig. 23.12 — Exercise 3, starting position. Key points: chin on chest; ankle on top of opposite knee.

ACTION

Bend forward using your lower back vertebrae. Allow your hands to fall *in front* of your shinbone. Reach downward with both hands as if you were going to try to touch your toes. Bend forward until you feel a good stretch (Fig. 23.13). You may feel the stretch in your lower back, your hip, buttock or your thigh. Stop and take stock of where you feel the restriction. Is your chin on your chest? Are you breathing freely and easily? Stay in this position until you feel that you have eased into it. Then, allow gravity to take you down a little bit farther toward your toes until you again feel a good stretch. Continue with this exercise until three minutes have passed. After three minutes, switch legs and repeat the above. Your *eventual* goal is to be able to reach your toes.

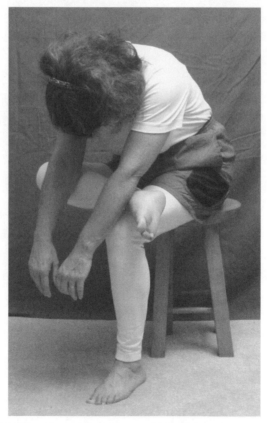

Fig. 23.13 — Exercise 3. Key points: chin on chest; bend forward at waist with arms in front of your leg.

ALTERNATIVE TO EXERCISE 3

STARTING POSITION

For those who are not able to bend their knees enough to cross the ankle onto the opposite knee *or* for those who have too much back pain or too big of a stomach when trying to bend forward at the waist, I suggest that you do the following alternative exercise. Lie on your back on the floor with your knees bent and your feet flat on the floor (Fig. 23.14).

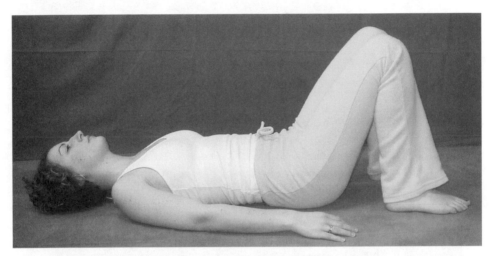

Fig. 23.14 — Alternative to Exercise 3, starting position. Lie flat on your back with knees bent and feet flat on floor.

ACTION

Start by lifting up one leg from the floor and bringing it toward you (start with the right leg). Place your right hand on the outside of the right knee and place your left hand around to the outside of the right ankle (Fig. 23.15). Lie back with your head on the floor. Then, using equal force with both arms, pull your leg toward your chest until you feel a good stretch in your hip, buttock, or along the back and side of your thigh (Fig. 23.16). Relax your shoulders as much as possible, but keep hold of the knee and ankle. Breathe freely and easily. Stay in this position until the stretching sensation eases. Then pull your leg closer to your chest until you again feel a good stretch. Repeat until three minutes have passed. Then switch legs and repeat the above. Your eventual goal is to be able to bring your leg as close to your chest as possible.

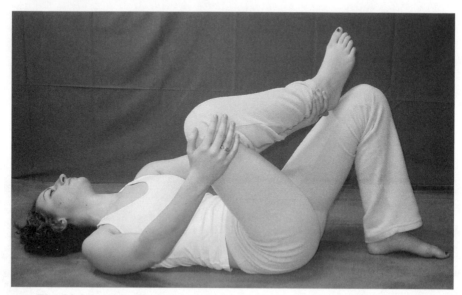

Fig. 23.15 — Alternative to Exercise 3. Key points: one hand on outside of ankle and the other hand on the outside of the knee.

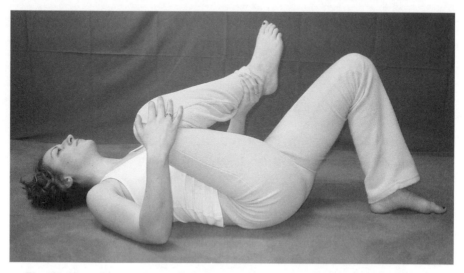

Fig. 23.16 — Alternative to Exercise 3. Key points: Keep your head on the floor, so as not to strain your neck. Using equal force with each arm, pull the leg, as one unit, toward your chest until you feel a good stretch.

SPECIAL EXERCISE FOR THOSE HAVING DIFFICULTY DOING EXERCISE 3

GENERAL

Some people are unable to do Exercise 3 because of their inability to externally rotate their hip joint. For example, when one tries to put the right ankle on top of the left knee, the right knee sticks up in the air instead of lying flat. Fig. 23.17 shows what a person looks like when (s)he is restricted in the ability to externally rotate the hip joint. If this photo reminds you of *yourself* when you try to do EXERCISE 3 above, you can improve your ability to open or externally rotate your hip joint by doing the following exercise.

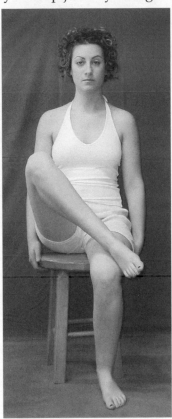

Fig. 23.17 — Special exercise for those having difficulty doing Exercise 3, explanation. For those who cannot do Exercise 3 because when they try, their knee sticks up in the air as in this photo. If this photo reminds you of you, I suggest the following exercises (see Fig. 23.18 and Fig. 23.19).

STARTING POSITION

Sit on the floor with your head and your lower back flat up against the wall. Bend your knees, place the **soles** of your feet together, and pull your feet as close to you as is comfortable. Place your hands on the insides of your knees (Fig. 23.18).

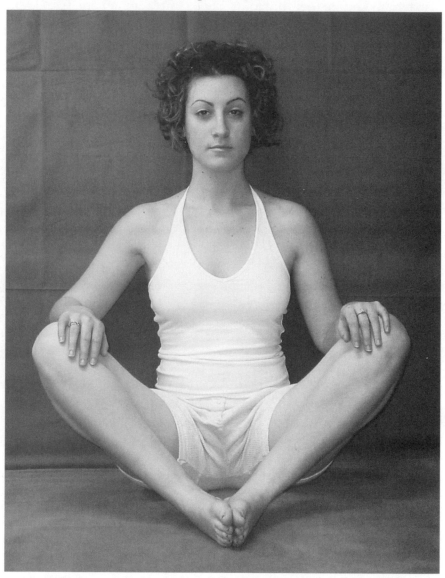

Fig. 23.18 — Special exercise for those having difficulty doing Exercise 3, starting position. Key points: entire spine and head flat up against the wall; soles of feet together; hands on the inside of the knees.

ACTION

Relax your entire body and gently push each knee down toward the floor until you feel a good stretch in the groin area and perineum (between your legs). Stop at this position. Breathe freely and easily. When you feel that you have relaxed into this position, gently push the knees down a little farther until you again feel a good stretch (Fig. 23.19). Repeat this until three minutes have passed. Your eventual goal is to be able to touch each knee to the floor. After you have done this exercise for a while and have increased your ability to externally rotate your hip, then go back and do EXERCISE 3 or the ALTERNATIVE TO EXERCISE 3.

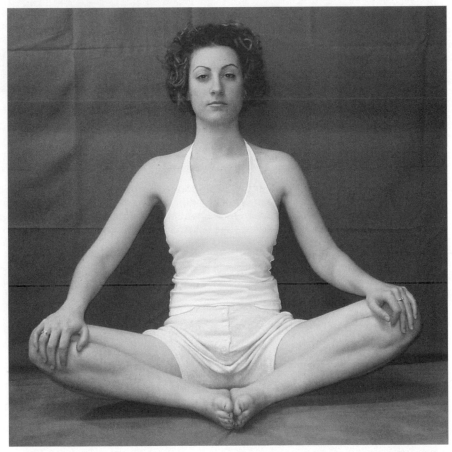

Fig. 23.19 — Special exercise for those having difficulty doing Exercise 3. Push your knees gently down toward the floor until you feel a good stretch in the groin area. Hold the stretch until the tightness releases and feels relaxed.

EXERCISE 4

STARTING POSITION

This exercise or posture is designed to increase the ability of your lower back to bend backwards. This is also called lumbar extension. Lie on the floor on your stomach. Place your *elbows together* on the floor in front of you with as much *separation* between your **elbows** and your **chest** as is comfortable. *Rest* your chin in your hands (Fig. 23.20).

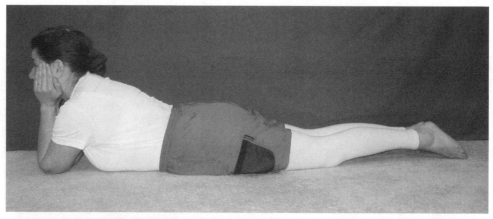

Fig. 23.20 — Exercise 4 is a posture designed to increase your ability to bend backwards (extend your lumbar spine). Key point: for maximum effect, keep elbows close together and as far away from your chest as possible. If too uncomfortable, this position can be modified (see Alternative to Exercise 4 in text).

ACTION

Lie in this position for a *maximum* of 5 minutes or as long as *comfortably* tolerated. Allow the lower back to relax and let your stomach sink into the floor. When you come out of this posture, first lie flat on your stomach, then roll onto either side and curl up into the fetal position and lie there for a few minutes before getting up (Fig. 23.21).

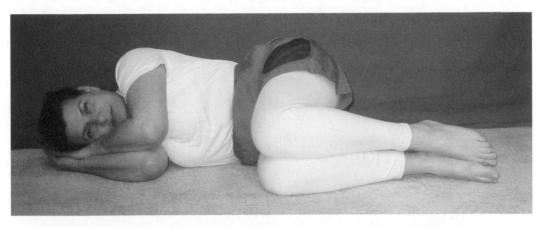

Fig. 23.21 — A resting posture after doing Exercise 4. Rest in this position for a few minutes before getting up, after having done Exercise 4.

ALTERNATIVE TO EXERCISE 4

STARTING POSITION

Some people may have difficulty doing EXERCISE 4 because lying in that position causes too much discomfort in the lower back and neck. For these people, I recommend lying on the floor on your stomach as if you were going to do EXERCISE 4 above. Then modify your position as follows:

1. Place a pillow under your belly.

2. Place your *elbows farther apart* than was described in EXERCISE 4 (Fig. 23.22) *or bring them close to your chest* (Fig. 23.22A). Then rest your chin in your hands.

    This position will put less strain on your lower back and neck.

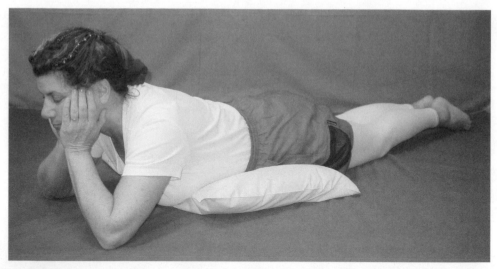

Fig. 23.22 — Alternative to Exercise 4, a modification. If Exercise 4 is too uncomfortable for your neck or lower back, place a pillow under your tummy and spread your elbows farther apart. This puts less strain on your neck and lower back.

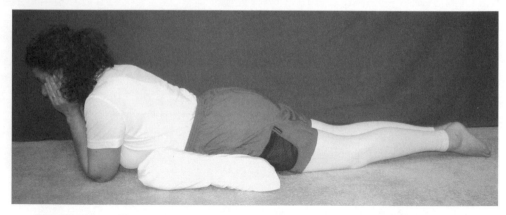

Fig. 23.22A — Alternative to Exercise 4, another modification. Simply bring your elbows as close to your chest a possible. This should also diminish any strain on your neck and lower back.

ACTION

Lie in this position for *up to* 5 minutes, as tolerated. Note that I said *up to* 5 minutes. Do it only for as long as you can be reasonably comfortable. An easy way to come out of this posture is to flatten out on the floor on your stomach. Then roll onto either side and curl up into the fetal position. Stay in the fetal position for a minute or so, then get up.

EXERCISE 5

STARTING POSITION

Lie on either side with your elbow on the floor and your head propped up on your hand (Fig. 23.23). Try to keep your body straight (keep your elbow and head in line with your trunk and legs).

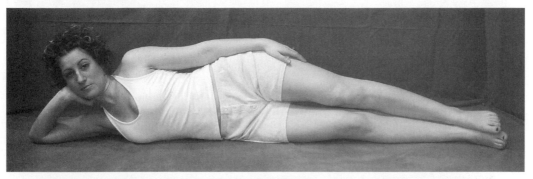

Fig. 23.23 — Exercise 5 is a posture designed to increase the ability of your spine to side-bend. Key point: keep your elbow and head in a straight line with your trunk and legs. Be sure to stretch both sides.

ACTION

Lie in this position for *up to* five minutes or as long as comfortably tolerated. After this exercise, lie on your back for 2-3 minutes before switching to stretch the other side.

ALTERNATIVE #1 TO EXERCISE 5

STARTING POSITION

Sometimes Exercise 5 can be uncomfortable, especially for persons who have restricted neck and/or shoulder motion. If this is the case, try this modification. Lie on your side with your elbow, forearm and hand as shown in Fig. 23.23A.

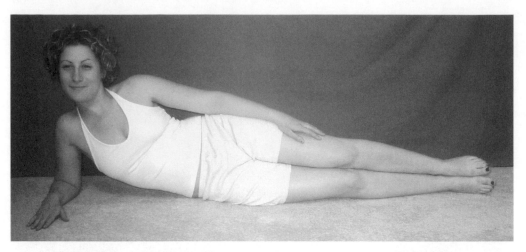

Fig. 23.23A — Alternative #1 to Exercise 5, starting position. Place elbow, forearm and hand as shown in this photo. Key point: allow your rib cage to "sink" toward the floor.

ACTION

Lie in this position for *up to* 5 minutes or as comfortably tolerated. You may find this a more comfortable position for your neck and shoulder. When finished, lie on your back for 2-3 minutes before switching to stretch the other side.

ALTERNATIVE #2 TO EXERCISE 5

STARTING POSITION

Some people may still find it difficult to perform the preceding two postures because of neck and/or shoulder discomfort. This simple, side-bending exercise will be easier. Stand up with feet shoulder-width apart and arms at your sides.

ACTION

Rest *either* forearm on top of your head and side-bend to the *opposite* side until you feel a good stretch (Fig. 23.23B). It's okay to let the neck side-bend also. You may feel the stretch from your neck down to your hip. Hold it for 15-30 seconds. Then, *slowly* come back to an upright position. Repeat the stretch 4 times. Remember to do the other side.

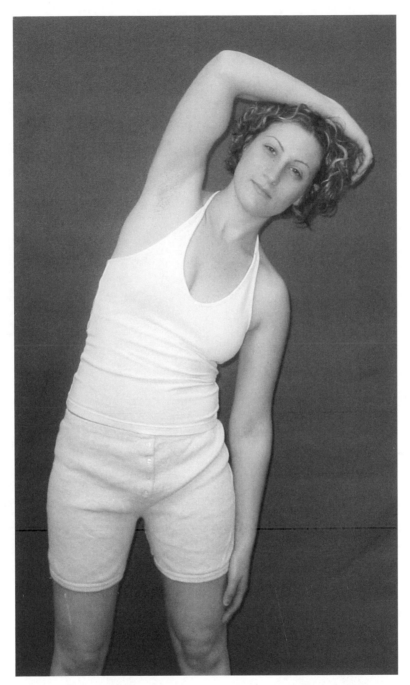

Fig. 23.23B — Alternative #2 to Exercise 5, action. This is an easier stretch, which will also increase your ability to side-bend. Hold the stretch for 15-30 seconds, then rest for a minute. Repeat the stretch 4 times. Then, side-bend to the opposite side.

EXERCISE 6

STARTING POSITION

Place your right knee on the floor (as shown in the photo) with your right hand on your right buttock (Fig. 23.24). Points to keep in mind:

- If this position is too uncomfortable for your knee, put a towel or a pillow under it.

- Flatten your tummy.

- Keep your lower back arched.

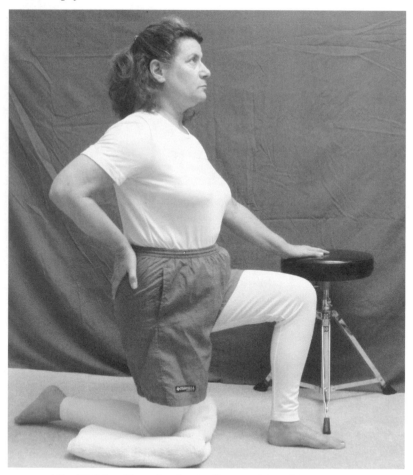

Fig. 23.24 — Exercise 6, starting position. Key points: keep lower back arched; hand on buttock.

ACTION

Tighten your buttocks. Keep them that way until the stretch is over. Keeping your back arched and, leading with your belly button, gently push your buttocks forward and slide your pelvis (hips) forward, "lunging" forward on your left leg (Fig. 23.25). You should feel a stretch in the front of your right hip and in your thigh. Hold this stretch for up to 30 seconds or as tolerated. Repeat this stretch three times. Then, switch to the other knee and repeat the above instructions to stretch the opposite side.

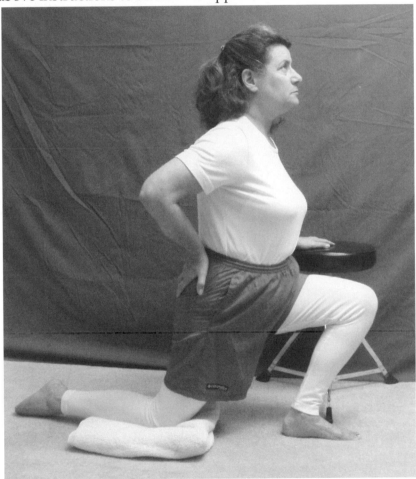

**Fig. 23.25 — Exercise 6. Key points: gently tighten buttocks; keep lower back arched; lead with your belly button and push your hips forward as you slowly "lunge" forward on your left leg. Hold for 15-30 seconds.
Then be sure to switch and do the other side.**

These are the exercises I do every day to stay flexible. Be careful, be regular, be persistent and be mindful as you do them. You will be amazed at how much more flexible you will become. These exercises, in conjunction with spinal manipulation, a lift (if needed) and muscle-balancing techniques, will be very helpful in relieving your lower back pain.

TWENTY-FOUR

Case Histories

Below are several case histories from my practice. I have included various clinical situations that you are likely to encounter.

CASE 1

SUBJECTIVE:

This man first came to my office at the age of 42. He had a 16-year history of recurrent, lower back pain and had been rejected by the military because of scoliosis (spinal curvature). The lower back pain was primarily left-sided and occasionally radiated down into the left leg. There was no history of numbness or weakness of the leg. He had been examined by an orthopedic surgeon and was told that his problem was not treatable with surgery. Physical therapy was also prescribed. Later in his search for relief, he went to an osteopath, with whom he treated for several years. Although his back would feel better for a while after spinal manipulation, the pain would return after only a few weeks.

OBJECTIVE:

Screening examination of the lower back showed that the right iliac crest was higher than the left. The greater trochanters (tops of the leg bones) were approximately equal in height. Because these findings suggested a pelvic tilt, UPRIGHT A-P and LATERAL x-rays were obtained and showed the following.

On the UPRIGHT A-P x-ray (Fig. 24.1), line AB connecting equal points on the sacral sulci (notches) shows that the right side of the pelvis is 23mm higher than the left. Note, also, that there is a lumbar scoliosis (curve) with the convexity "bulging" in the direction of the lower (left) side of the pelvis. In this x-ray, please note that the legs are *equal* in length (line GH).

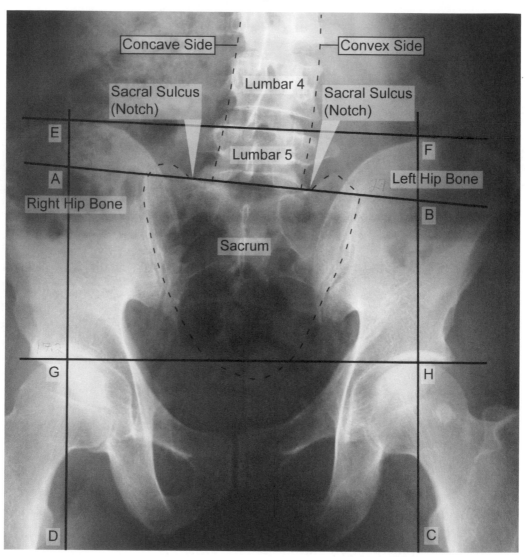

Fig. 24.1 — Shows right side of pelvis higher than left by 23mm at the sacral sulci (notches) (line AB). Legs are equal length (line GH). Lumbar scoliosis is convex (bulging) left.

Measurement and analysis of the UPRIGHT LATERAL x-ray (Fig. 24.2) shows the sacral base angle to be 26-degrees (small sacral base angle). The perpendicular line (EF), dropped from the middle of the body of L3, passes through the body of S1. Notice how straight the lumbar spine is on this **side view**. Therefore, there is no concern about too much lumbar lordosis when prescribing the lift because this person has hardly any lordosis at all.

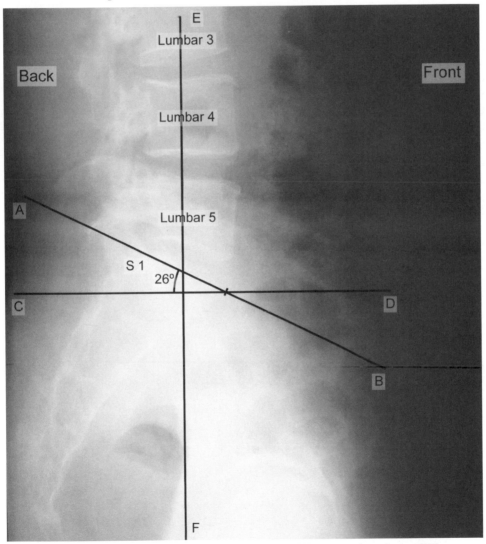

Fig. 24.2 — Shows a small sacral base angle (26 degrees) and very little lumbar lordosis. Line EF passes through the body of S1. This person would benefit greatly from lumbar extension exercises.

ASSESSMENT:

#1. Lumbosacral strain. #2. Pelvic tilt. #3. Lumbar scoliosis. #4. Diminished lumbar lordosis.

PLAN:

The lumbar spine and pelvic biomechanics were evaluated and treated with spinal manipulation. After a few treatments, lift therapy was begun with a 1/4-inch lift for the left shoe. The patient was treated with manual medicine (manipulation) and stretching exercises. He was clinically evaluated at each visit. After three months of weekly visits, the patient reported he was feeling much better. The final lift prescription turned out to be 1/2-inch, based upon the fact that the patient was feeling well and upon the presence of free and easy biomechanical motion of the lumbar spine and pelvis. Remember: you *don't have to* give the entire prescription if the patient feels well and good biomechanical motion has been restored.

COMMENT:

With such a small sacral base angle and demonstrating very little lumbar lordosis on the upright lateral x-ray, this person would benefit greatly from doing lumbar extension exercises (see Chapter Twenty-Three, EXERCISE 4).

CASE 2

SUBJECTIVE:

This 66-year old man was a retired construction worker who injured his lower back during the course of many years of hard work and heavy lifting. The patient had been treated with chiropractic manipulation on many occasions with only temporary relief. The pain gradually worsened to the point where he had bilateral leg pain and right leg numbness. He saw an orthopedic surgeon who requested a Magnetic Resonance Imaging (MRI) scan, which revealed a protruding disc at L5-S1. He was scheduled for surgery which he postponed in order to try "cortisone injections" as a last effort to avoid surgery. The injections failed to give him relief. Four months he came to my office.

OBJECTIVE:

The screening examination of the lower back showed the left iliac crest and left greater trochanter were higher than those on the right. Because of the inequality of the iliac crests and greater trochanters, UPRIGHT A-P AND LATERAL x-rays of the pelvis were taken. The x-rays reveal the following: on the A-P view, the left side of the pelvis is 20mm higher than the right at the sacral sulci (notches) (Fig. 24.3, line AB). The left leg is only 4mm longer than the right (line GH). There is a lumbar scoliosis with a convexity (bulging) toward the lower (right) side of the pelvis.

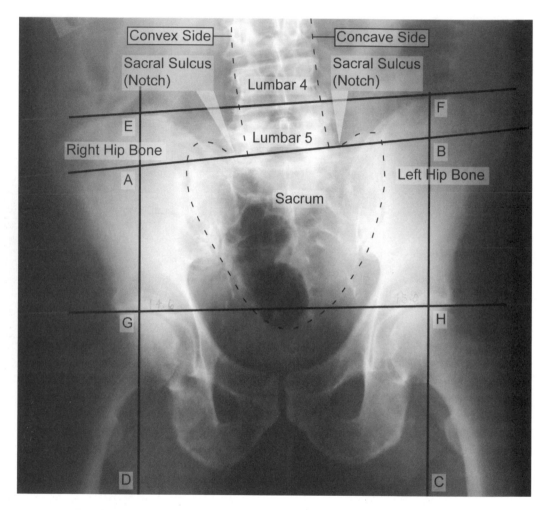

Fig. 24.3 — A-P upright of the pelvis shows the left side of the pelvis is higher than the right side by 20mm at the sacral sulci (line AB). The left leg is only 4mm longer than the right (line GH). Lumbar scoliosis (curve) is convex (bulging) toward the lower (right) side of the pelvis.

The LATERAL view (Fig. 24.4) shows a sacral base angle of 41-degrees. Line EF, from the midpoint of the body of L3, passes through the body of S1.

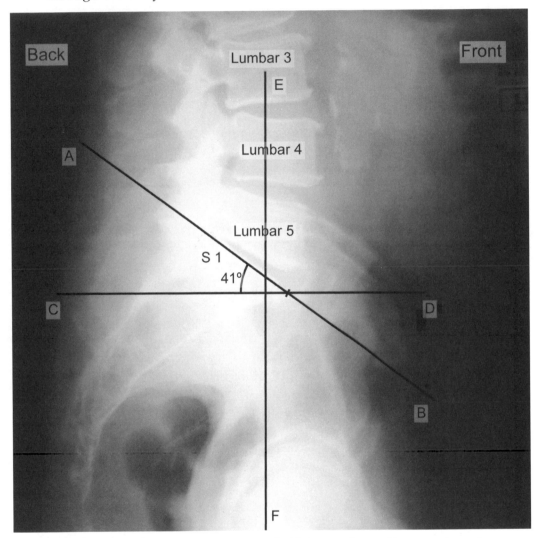

Fig. 24.4 — Upright lateral shows a normal (41 degrees) sacral base angle and a normal degree of lumbar lordosis (line EF passes through the body of S1).

ASSESSMENT:

#1. Chronic lumbosacral strain. #2. Pelvic tilt. #3. Lumbar scoliosis. #4. Protrusion L5 disk with radiculopathy.

PLAN:

The patient was started on a 7mm lift for the right shoe. The patient was seen weekly for four consecutive weeks. With each visit, he continued to improve. He said the lift seemed to make a great difference. At the end of the fourth visit, he said he was going on a fishing vacation for a few months and would schedule another visit upon his return. This was in February 2001. Because I had not heard anything from him since his last visit (six months previously), I telephoned him, just prior to the writing of this book, to find out how he was doing. He said that his lower back pain has not been a problem since the last time I saw him. He wears the lift and does his exercises every day.

COMMENT:

This man exhibited three of the six frequent causes of failed lower back syndrome: pelvic tilt, a flexed lumbar vertebra and a posterior nutation of the sacrum. Even though this patient had a protruding disk as demonstrated on the MRI, it was not the cause of his pain.

With a pelvic tilt of 20mm, I would have preferred to have the patient wear at least a 1/2-inch (12-13mm) lift as a total lift prescription. However, it's hard to argue with success. You will often be amazed at how little lift correction is required to give lasting relief to the patient. If the patient comes in again, I will certainly make sure he has free and easy biomechanical motion in the lumbar spine and pelvis. If not, I will prescribe a larger lift. But for the time being, he was feeling great and was off on *another* extended fishing vacation.

CASE 3

SUBJECTIVE:

This 48-year old woman fell 14 years ago and landed on her buttocks, resulting in a fracture of her "tailbone." Since that time, she had left-side lower back pain. Over this 14-year period she had been treated conventionally by her medical doctor and, subsequently, received manipulation from an osteopath, a chiropractor, and a naturopathic physician. She also had extensive physical therapy, yet she still had constant low back pain.

OBJECTIVE:

Screening examination of the lower back showed the right iliac crest to be higher than the left. The height of the greater trochanters appeared equal. Looking at the A-P UPRIGHT x-ray (Fig. 24.5), we can see that the right side of the pelvis higher than the left by a difference of 21mm (approx. 7/8-inch) at the sacral sulci (notches) (line AB). Also, there is a lumbar scoliosis with the convexity toward the lower (left) side of the pelvis and the legs are the same length (line GH).

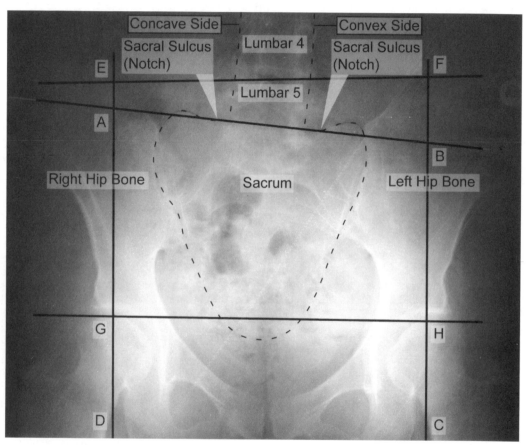

Fig. 24.5 — Upright A-P x-ray shows the right side of the pelvis higher than the left by 21mm at the sacral sulci (notches) (line AB) , however, the legs are the same length (line GH). There is a lumbar scoliosis (curve) with the convexity toward the lower (left) side of the pelvis.

The UPRIGHT LATERAL x-ray (Fig. 24.6) shows that the sacral base angle is *50-degrees* and that the perpendicular line (EF) from the middle of the body of L3 passes **anterior** to (in front of) the body of S1. This means that the patient has an increased amount of lumbar lordosis or "sway back." Therefore, care must be taken as to how to apply the lift (Chapter Eighteen).

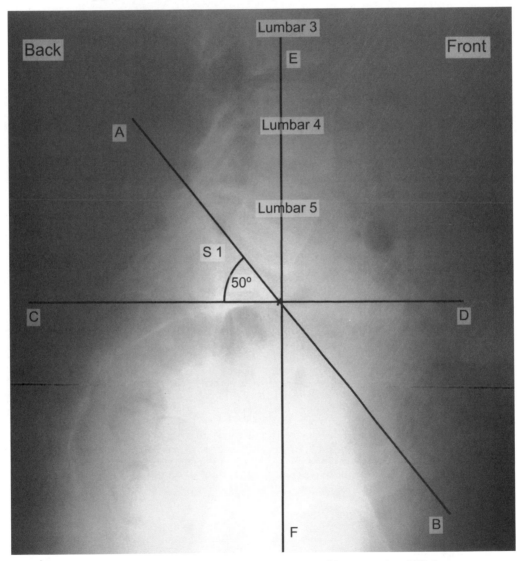

Fig. 24.6 — The upright lateral x-ray shows a sacral base angle of 50 degrees and line EF passes in front of the body of S1, indicating a exaggerated amount of lumbar lordosis (sway back).

ASSESSMENT:

#1. Chronic lumbosacral strain. #2. Pelvic tilt. #3. Exaggerated lumbar lordosis.

PLAN:

Manual medicine techniques (manipulation) were applied to the lumbar spine and pelvis to restore free and easy biomechanical motion. A stretching exercise program was prescribed for the patient to do at home and a 1/4-inch lift was prescribed for the inside of the left shoe. The patient was seen once weekly for one month when the lumbar spine and pelvis were evaluated and treated. After one month, the lift size was increased to 3/8-inch inside the left shoe. The patient tolerated this well and reported that she felt much better. She was able to do her daily activities with little or no pain.

The final lift height that brought complete relief to this patient and allowed free and easy motion of the lumbar spine and pelvis was 1/2-inch. This was prescribed as follows: 1/4-inch was applied to the entire sole of the left shoe and an additional 1/4-inch was added just to the heel of the left shoe to minimize the strain on an already exaggerated lumbar lordosis (see Chapter Eighteen).

COMMENT:

This patient exhibited three of the six causes of a failed lower back syndrome: shear dysfunction of the innominate (hip) bone, pubic symphysis dysfunction and pelvic tilt.

CASE 4

SUBJECTIVE:

This 49-year old woman had a seven-year history of low back pain, worse on the right side. The pain went down into the right lower extremity and, at times, the leg would "give out" due to sudden pain. She had been treated by a chiropractor for several years, who had prescribed a 1/2-inch lift to be worn in the right shoe. The patient continued to have pain in spite of the lift.

OBJECTIVE:

The screening examination of the lower back showed the left iliac crest and the left greater trochanter higher than the right. The A-P UPRIGHT x-ray (Fig. 24.7), taken when the patient was barefoot, shows the left side of the pelvis to be *33mm* higher than the right at the sacral sulci (notches) (line AB). That is a lot of tilt. The left leg is 15mm longer than the right (line GH). There is a lumbar scoliosis with the convexity (bulge) toward the lower (right) side of the pelvis.

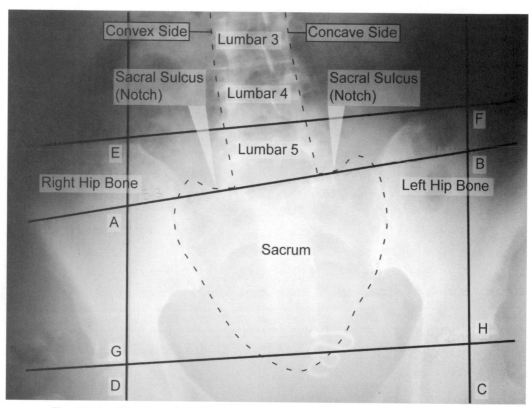

Fig. 24.7 — Standing, barefoot, upright x-ray of pelvis shows the left side of the pelvis higher than the right by 33mm at the sacral sulci (notches) (line AB). The left leg is 15mm longer than the right (line GH). The lumbar scoliosis (curve) is convex (bulging) to the right.

The UPRIGHT LATERAL x-ray (Fig. 24.8) shows increased lumbar lordosis with a sacral base angle of 48 degrees. The perpendicular line (EF) from the middle of the body of L3 passes anterior to (in front of) the body of S1, indicating exaggerated lumbar lordosis.

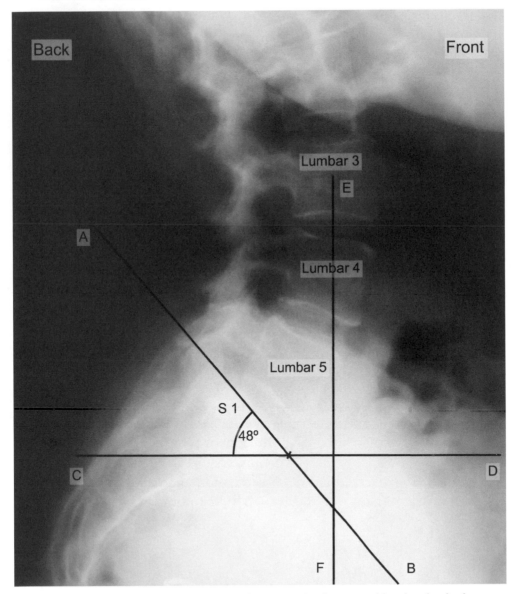

Fig. 24.8 — The upright lateral x-ray demonstrates increased lumbar lordosis with a sacral base angle of 48 degrees with line EF passing anterior to (in front of) the body of S1.

ASSESSMENT:

#1. Chronic lumbosacral strain. #2. Marked pelvic tilt with exaggerated lumbar lordosis. #3. Lumbar scoliosis.

PLAN:

Because the patient was already wearing a 1/2-inch lift and was still having back pain, the lift prescription was ultimately increased to a full inch, divided between the heel and the sole (as discussed in Chapter Eighteen). The patient was also treated with spinal manipulation on a weekly basis as well as muscle balancing and stretching exercises for 3-4 months, helping her to adapt to the very large lift prescription. The patient now enjoys a pain-free lower back that has good biomechanical motion.

COMMENT:

This patient had three of the six causes of a failed lower back: pelvic tilt, pubic symphysis dysfunction and muscle imbalance of the trunk and lower extremities.

ADDENDUM:

Several months after completion of therapy, another A-P UPRIGHT x-ray (Fig. 24.9) was taken of this patient, this time with her shoes on and her lift in place. This x-ray shows the difference between the two sides of the pelvis is now 7mm (left greater than right), instead of 33mm (line AB). Also, notice that her right leg now appears "longer" than her left leg due to the 25mm lift built onto the bottom of the right shoe (line GH). Remember, leg length by itself doesn't matter in the treatment of pelvic tilt. In this patient, the fact that she always wore Birkenstock sandals—which have a "negative heel"—made it a lot easier for her to tolerate such a large lift with her already exaggerated lumbar lordosis.

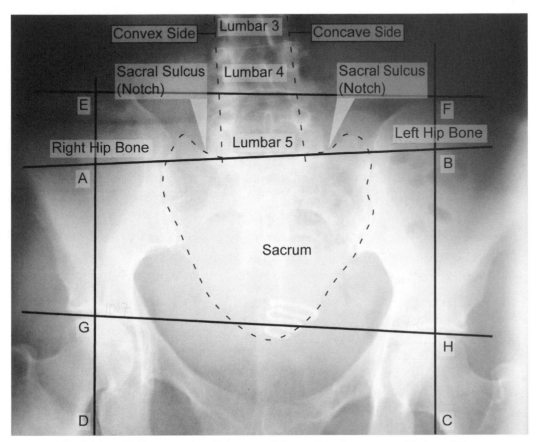

Fig. 24.9 — Follow-up standing x-ray, taken with shoes on and 25mm lift on right shoe. Notice the left side of the pelvis is now only 7mm higher than the right (line AB). Note the right leg is now "longer" than the left because of the large amount of lift correction required for the right shoe (line GH). Remember, we're treating pelvic tilt, not leg length. Also, please see that there has been a reduction in the amount of lumbar scoliosis (curve) when compared with Fig. 24.7.

CASE 5

SUBJECTIVE:

This 27-year old woman had a five-year history of lower back pain that began after an automobile accident. Prior to the accident she had been quite athletic (long distance running). After recovering from the accident, she tried to resume her training for a marathon race but was unable to do so because of right lower back pain. There was no involvement of the lower extremities. She had gone to a licensed massage therapist for a period of two years, but this offered only temporary relief. Other than massage, she had no other therapy for a year before coming to my office.

OBJECTIVE:

The screening examination of the lower back showed the left iliac crest higher than the right. The greater trochanters were approximately the same height. The A-P UPRIGHT x-ray (Fig. 24.10) shows the left side of the pelvis higher than the right by 7mm at the sacral base (line AB). The legs are the same length (line GH). There is a lumbar scoliosis with the convexity (bulging) toward the lower (right) side of the pelvis.

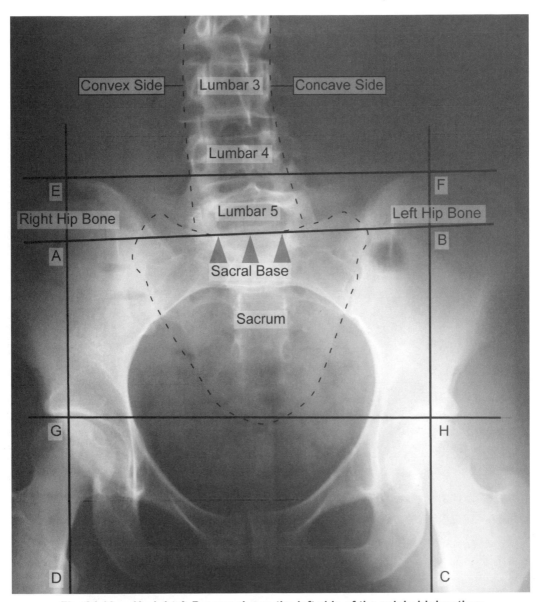

Fig. 24.10 — Upright A-P x-ray shows the left side of the pelvis higher than the right by 7mm at the sacral base (line AB). The legs are the same length (line GH). There is a lumbar scoliosis (curve) with the convexity to the lower (right) side.

The UPRIGHT LATERAL x-ray (Fig. 24.11) shows an increased lumbar lordosis characterized by a sacral base angle of *54 degrees*, and that line EF, from the middle of the body of L3, passes anterior to (in front of) the body of S1.

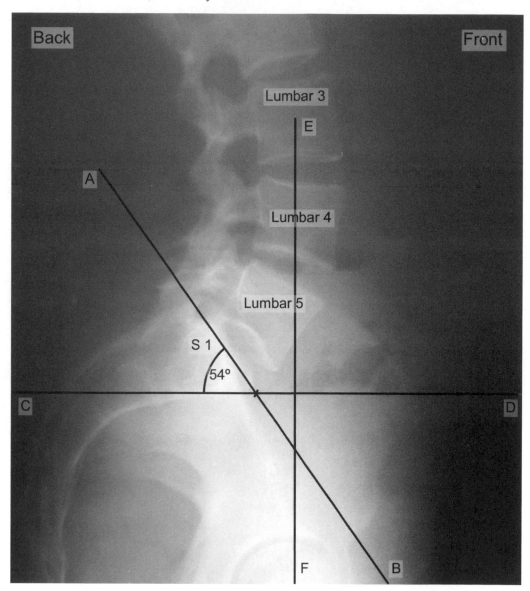

Fig. 24.11 — The upright lateral shows an increased amount of lumbar lordosis with a sacral base angle of 54 degrees and with line EF passing well in front of the body of S1.

ASSESSMENT:

#1. Chronic lumbosacral strain. #2. Pelvic tilt with increased lumbar lordosis. #3. Lumbar scoliosis.

PLAN:

Spinal manipulation was begun in order to restore free and easy biomechanical motion to the lumbar spine and pelvis. A 6mm lift was applied to the inside of the right shoe and exercises were given to restore muscle balance to the trunk and extremities. The patient was treated seven times over the next three months. She has been symptom free as of the writing of this book (several months later).

COMMENT:

This patient exhibited four of the six causes of a failed lower back syndrome: Pelvic tilt, muscle imbalance of the trunk and lower extremities, posterior nutation of the sacrum and a flexed lumbar vertebra.

CASE 6

SUBJECTIVE

This 78-year old man had a 25 year history of intermittent lower back pain. About one year prior to his first visit to my office, the lower back pain became worse and began to radiate down into his right leg. The pain became so severe that, for a few weeks, he had to use a wheelchair to get around. The patient also complained of numbness and tingling of the right leg, from the knee down to the foot.

He was evaluated by his primary care physician, who made a diagnosis of peripheral neuropathy. He was placed on Neurontin, a medication often used for nerve pain and a narcotic pain medication called oxycodone. He was then referred to a neurosurgeon who requested a Magnetic Resonance Imaging (MRI) scan. The scan showed that, between L4 and L5, a piece of the disk between the two vertebrae had broken off and was *possibly* irritating the nerve root. According to the patient, the neurosurgeon did not want to operate at that time.

OBJECTIVE:

Screening examination of the lower back showed the left iliac crest and the left greater trochanter higher than the right. The UPRIGHT A-P x-ray (Fig. 24.12) shows that the left side of the pelvis is 6mm higher than the right at the sacral sulci (notches) (line AB). The left leg is 12mm longer than the right (line GH). There is a lumbar scoliosis with the convexity (bulge) toward the lower (right) side of the pelvis.

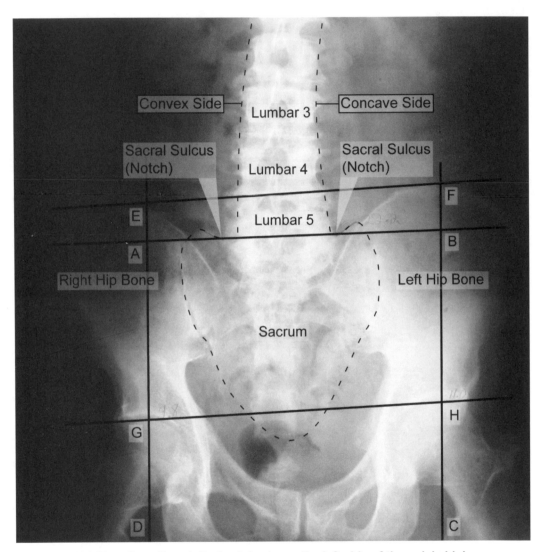

Fig. 24.12 — Standing, A-P of pelvis shows the left side of the pelvis higher than the right by 6mm at the sacral sulci (notches) (line AB). The left leg, however, is 12mm longer than the right (line GH). There is a lumbar scoliosis (curve) with the convexity to the right.

A look at the UPRIGHT LATERAL x-ray (see Fig. 24.13), shows that the sacral base angle measures 30-degrees and that line EF, drawn the middle of the body of L3, passes through the body of S1. Note that the patient has very little lumbar lordosis (curve).

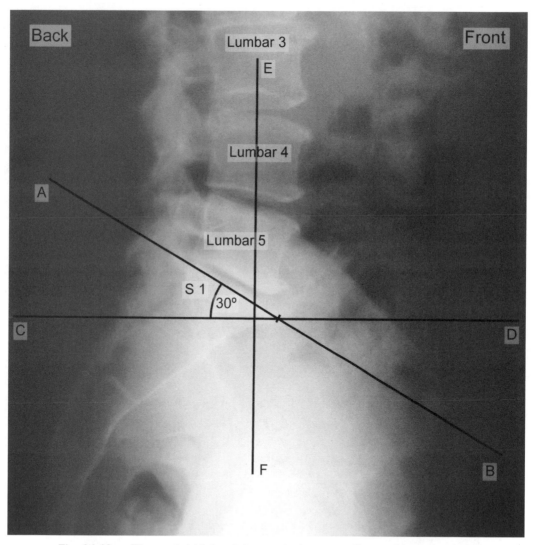

Fig. 24.13 — The upright lateral demonstrates a small sacral base angle (30 degrees). There is very little lumbar lordosis (sway back). In fact, the lower lumbar spine is almost "flat". Line EF passes through the body of S1. This person would greatly benefit from lumbar extension exercise (Chapter Twenty-Three EXERCISE 4).

ASSESSMENT:

#1. Focal disk extrusion L4-5, paracentral and lateral on the right with extrusion of disk material into the lateral recess of L5, probably affecting the L5 nerve root (from the MRI). #2. Chronic lumbosacral strain. #3. Pelvic tilt. #4. Lumbar scoliosis.

PLAN:

Spinal manipulation was begun to restore free and easy motion to the lumbar spine and pelvis. A 1/4-inch lift was prescribed to wear inside the right shoe. Exercises were prescribed to stretch and balance the muscles of the trunk and extremities. After two months of weekly manipulative treatment, doing the exercises and wearing the lift, the patient said he was 90% improved. He had stopped using the medications that he was taking. The numbness in his leg had disappeared completely. After another month, the patient was discharged to return as needed. He is enjoying a pain-free, normal life again.

COMMENT:

This patient had four of the six causes of a failed lower back syndrome: a pelvic tilt, muscle imbalance of the trunk and lower extremities, a flexed lumbar vertebra, and a posterior sacral torsion. Further, with such a small sacral base angle and almost no lumbar lordosis, this patient benefited greatly from lumbar extension exercises (see Chapter Twenty-Three, EXERCISE 4).

CASE 7

SUBJECTIVE:

This 21-year old woman presented with a history of intermittent right lower back pain for the previous six months. The pain started after having lifted a heavy box and turning to place it on a counter. The pain was aggravated by sitting. A few months of massage therapy didn't seem to make any long-term difference. One day at work, her entire right leg went numb. This frightened her and she made an appointment to see me.

OBJECTIVE:

The screening examination of the lower back showed left iliac crest higher than the right. The greater trochanters were approximately of equal height. The A-P UPRIGHT x-ray (Fig. 24.14) shows the left side of the pelvis higher than the right by 8mm at the sacral sulci (notches) (line AB). The legs are of equal length (line GH). There is a very slight lumbar curve with the convexity (bulging) toward the lower (right) side of the pelvis.

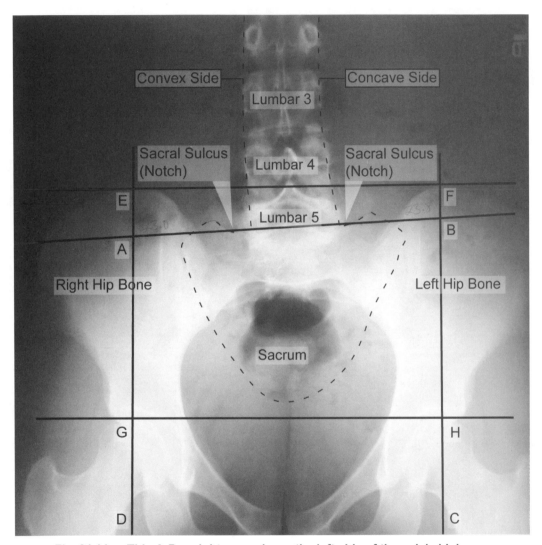

Fig. 24.14 — This A-P upright x-ray shows the left side of the pelvis higher than the right by 8mm at the sacral sulci (notches) (line AB). The legs are equal in length (line GH). The slight scoliosis is convex to the lower (right) side of the pelvis.

The LATERAL UPRIGHT x-ray (Fig. 24.15) shows an exaggerated lumbar lordosis with a sacral base angle of *64-degrees*. Line EF, drawn from the middle of the body of L3, passes well anterior to (in front of) the body of S1.

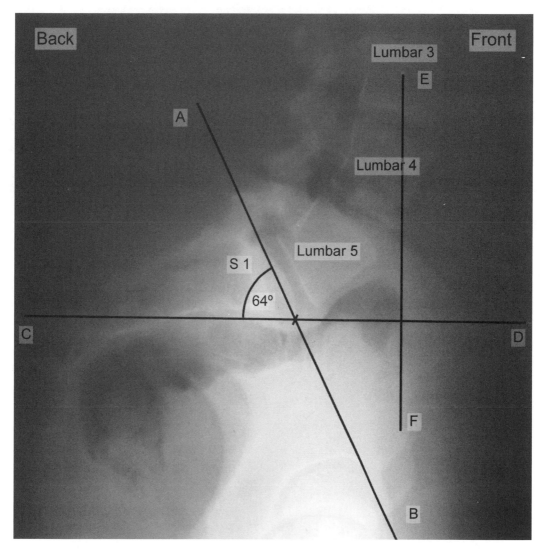

Fig. 24.15 — The upright lateral shows a very large sacral base angle of 64 degrees. Line EF passes well anterior to the body of S1. This represents a very large amount of lumbar lordosis.

ASSESSMENT:

#1. Chronic, lumbosacral strain. #2. Pelvic tilt. #3. Exagerated lumbar lordosis.

PLAN:

Manual medicine techniques were applied and an 8mm lift was prescribed for the inside of the right shoe. Because the patient was so young and flexible, she was able to tolerate it without any difficulty, even with the exaggerated lumbar lordosis. In addition to manipulation and the lift, stretching and muscle balancing exercises were prescribed to restore free and easy biomechanical motion to the lumbar spine and pelvis. The patient had three treatments before the low back pain disappeared. She has continued to wear her lift, do her exercises, and to feel well.

COMMENT:

This patient had four of the six causes of a failed lower back syndrome: pelvic tilt, muscle imbalance of the trunk and lower extremities, a flexed lumbar vertebra and a posterior sacral torsion.

CASE 8

SUBJECTIVE:

This 40-year old woman did hard, physical labor for her livelihood. She had injured herself moving or lifting something very heavy on three separate occasions. She had been evaluated and treated by at least two different chiropractors over a period of six or seven years. One of the chiropractors prescribed a 1/8-inch lift. However, *no x-rays* were taken before the lift was prescribed. The relief that she obtained from all of her previous therapies was at best temporary. She then came to see me.

At the time of the first visit, she complained of left low back pain, left hip, and left buttock pain. There was no leg pain, no numbness and no weakness present.

OBJECTIVE:

The screening examination of the lower back showed that the right iliac crest and right greater trochanter were higher than the left. A-P and LATERAL UPRIGHT x-rays of the pelvis were taken. The A-P UPRIGHT (Fig. 24.16) demonstrates the right side of the pelvis higher than the left by *30mm* at the sacral base (line AB). The right leg is longer than the left by 11mm (line GH). A mild lumbar scoliosis is present with the convexity (bulge) toward the lower (left) side of the pelvis.

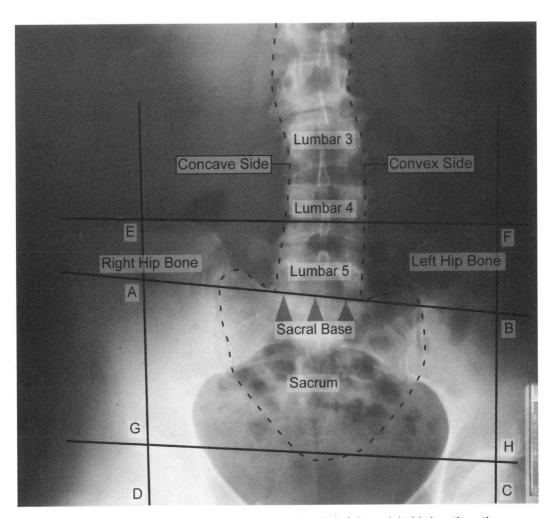

Fig. 24.16 — The A-P upright shows the right side of the pelvis higher than the left by 30mm at the sacral base (line AB). The right leg is longer than the left by 11mm (line GH). There is a lumbar scoliosis that is convex to the left.

The LATERAL UPRIGHT x-ray shows a sacral base angle of 37-degrees (Fig. 24.17). The perpendicular line (EF), from the middle of the body of L3, passes through the body of S1.

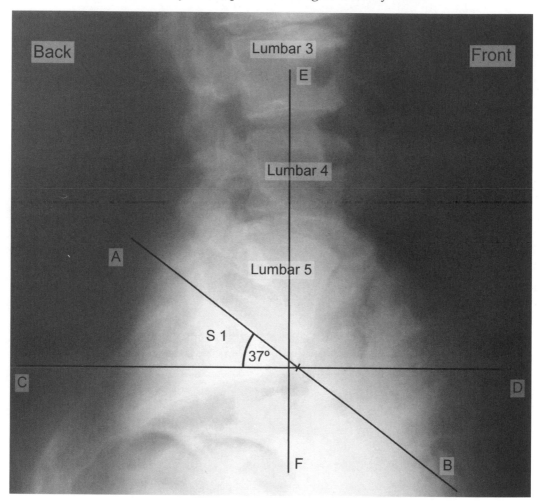

Fig. 24.17 — The upright lateral x-ray shows a slightly smaller than normal sacral base angle (37 degrees). Line EF passes through the body of S1.

ASSESSMENT:

#1. Chronic, lumbosacral strain. #2. Pelvic tilt. #3. Lumbar scoliosis.

PLAN:

This patient presented some significant challenges to treatment. First, she did hard physical labor on a daily basis and could not afford to lose her job. Second, she had very tight muscles. Third, she had a large amount pelvic tilt. However she was very motivated to get better. She was prescribed a 1/4-inch lift to be worn inside of the left shoe. Stretching and muscle balancing exercises were also prescribed. She was seen once weekly for evaluation and manipulation. After two months, the lift was increased to 1/2-inch to be worn inside of the left shoe. She was able to tolerate this well because she did her exercises twice daily.

After four months, the lift was again increased to 3/4-inch. This was applied by adding 3/8-inch to the entire sole of the left shoe and an additional 3/8-inch lift to the heel of the same shoe. The lifts that she had been wearing inside the shoe were discontinued.

After one month of wearing the 3/4-inch lift (five months after having begun treatment), the patient was 75 percent improved with respect to lower back pain. At the end of the sixth month of weekly treatment, the patient was able to reduce the number of treatments to three per month. After one year of treatment, the patient's clinical condition improved dramatically. She subsequently began to come in on an "as needed" basis. I now see her for an "adjustment" about two to three times per year. She works full-time and took up body-building.

COMMENT:

This patient had two of the six causes of a failed lower back: pelvic tilt and muscle imbalance of the trunk and lower extremities. This example is to encourage you not to give up if the patient does not improve right away. Follow the patient closely. Apply the principles of lift prescription. Make sure the patient is doing the exercises regularly and correctly. Sometimes it just takes time. Everybody gets better at his/her own pace.

CASE 9

SUBJECTIVE

A 49-year old man had a ten-year history of constant, sharp, lower back pain, that had become much worse over the previous five years. He had been an avid cyclist and cross-country skier, but had to give these up due to constant lower back pain. The pain was mostly in the right lower back with no radiation into the lower extremity. There was no numbness or weakness present. He had been evaluated and treated by his primary care physician, a sports medicine physician and an orthopedic surgeon. Although the patient had several months of physical therapy with someone skilled in spinal manipulation and muscle-balancing techniques, he still had constant lower back pain.

OBJECTIVE

The screening examination of the lower back showed that the left iliac crest and the greater trochanter were higher than the right. The UPRIGHT A-P x-ray (Fig. 24.18) shows the left side of the pelvis higher than the right by 18mm at the sacral base (line AB). The left leg is 8mm longer than the right (line GH). There is a mild lumbar scoliosis with the convexity (bulge) to the right.

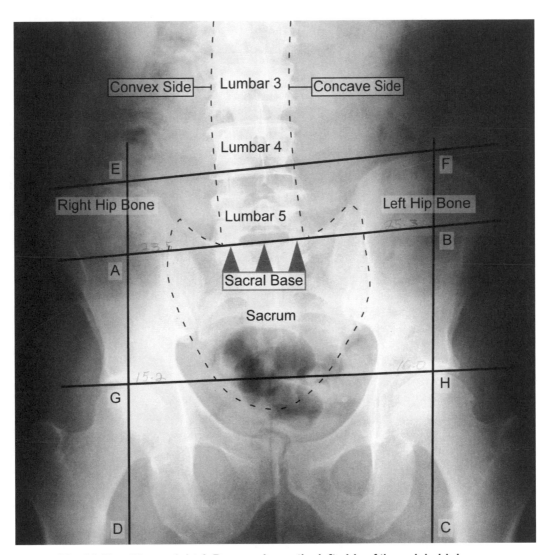

Fig. 24.18 — The upright A-P x-ray shows the left side of the pelvis higher than the right by 18mm at the sacral base (line AB). The left leg is 8mm longer than the right (line GH). The lumbar curve is convex (bulging) to the right.

The UPRIGHT LATERAL x-ray (Fig. 24.19) shows a sacral base angle of almost 34 degrees. The perpendicular line (EF), from the middle of the body of L3, passes through the posterior aspect (back) of the body of S1. Excessive lumbar lordosis is *not* a factor.

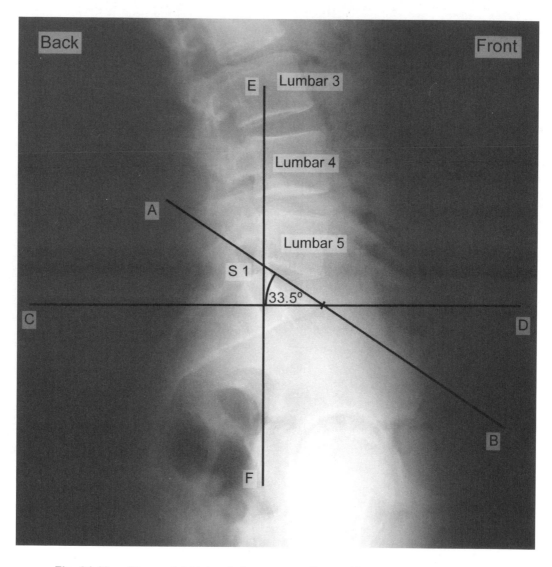

Fig. 24.19 — The upright lateral shows a small sacral base angle of 33.5 degrees and line EF passes through the most posterior (very back) part of the body of S1. This indicates that the person would greatly benefit from lumbar extension exercises (chapter twenty-three, EXERCISE 4).

ASSESSMENT

#1. Chronic lumbosacral strain. #2. Pelvic tilt. #3. Lumbar scoliosis.

PLAN

Spinal manipulation was begun in order to restore free and easy motion of the lumbar spine and pelvis. A 3/8-inch lift was prescribed for the inside the right boot (the patient wore boots most of the time). Stretching exercises were demonstrated for the patient to do at home. The patient was seen once weekly. At the first few treatment sessions, the exercises were reviewed in detail, the patient was examined and spinal manipulation was performed. After the third visit, the patient said that the sharp pain was gone from his lower back.

Although the patient was feeling better after one month, the lift was increased from 3/8-inch (9-10mm) to 14mm because my examination did not demonstrate free and easy motion of the lumbar spine and pelvis. The lift was applied as follows: one half of the lift prescription (7mm) was applied to the entire sole of the right boot and the other half of the lift prescription (7mm) was applied to just the heel of the same boot.

Two and one-half months after the beginning of treatment, the patient reported a pain free lower back. I wish you could see the smile on his face.

COMMENT

This patient had three of the six causes of a failed lower back syndrome: pelvic tilt, a flexed lumbar vertebrae and a posterior nutation of the sacrum. With such a small sacral base angle and the fact that line EF passes through the very back part of the body of S1, this person would greatly benefit from lumbar extension exercises (Chapter Twenty-Three, EXERCISE 4)

The Last Chapter

Well, dear reader, this has been a labor of love for me. I have done my best to explain to you, as simply as I can, how to find out if you have a pelvic tilt and what to do about it. I know that there were lots of new things to learn, especially for those of you who are not health care professionals. However, I have always had the *greatest confidence* in the ability of my patients to understand their medical problems and to participate successfully in their own treatment. I know that with what you have learned, you can take over from this point and carry things to a successful outcome. Be patient and persistent. I wish you good luck.

When I was a sophomore medical student, one of the courses we had to take before beginning our "clinical" years was called "physical diagnosis." The course was taught by a physician named Nathan Galloway, M.D. In the course, I learned how to take a medical history and to do a physical examination. I thought that this course was the "heart and soul" of medicine. I also thought that if I could just learn to do a thorough physical examination then I would be a good physician. In other words, I thought that the physical examination was much more important than the patient's history. This is not so. Dr. Galloway said something I will never forget. He said, "*Listen* to the patient. (S)he's *telling* you what's wrong." He was absolutely right. The key to being a good physician is being a good listener.

To my esteemed health care professional colleagues, with whom I am proud to be associated, I respectfully ask this of you:

please listen to your patients with chronic or recurrent low back pain. Listen for the clues: the *one-sided* low back pain, the not-uncommon *radiation* into the buttock, thigh or leg, the *recurrent nature* of the symptoms over several months or years, the *many visits* to *many HCPs*, the *lack of findings* indicating surgery and the *inability* of the patient to get relief. In short, listen for the **Humpty Dumpty Syndrome.**

I know how busy you are. I know what it's like to have a patient with chronic low back pain walk into the office on a day when the schedule is full and the waiting room is packed. Writing a prescription or sending the patient to physical therapy is easy. However, if you will invest some time to learn and apply the simple method outlined in this book, you will be amazed at how many of your patients you will help. People who thought they were going to have to live with their lower back pain for the rest of their lives will instead be grateful to you for the rest of their lives.

Humpty Dumpty sat on a wall
Humpty Dumpty had a great fall
All the kings horses and all the kings men.....
CAN put Humpty Dumpty together again.

INDEX

Additional copies of *THE HUMPTY DUMPTY SYNDROME* are available from:

MASTER'S PLAN PUBLISHING L.L.C.
2727 NW Ninth Street
Corvallis, OR 97330

Phone Orders: 541-758-3456
Fax Orders: 541-757-8250
E-Mail: mastersplanpublishing@earthlink.net
Website: http://www.mastersplanpublishing.com

$23.95 for each copy, plus $4.00 shipping and handling for first copy ($2.00 each additional copy).